MW00948204

OUT *of* OBESITY
AND INTO THE PROMISED LAND

A Personal Journey from Obesity to
Weight Loss Surgery Success

JULIA HOLLOMAN

Text, Concept and Design: Copyright © 2014 by
Julia Holloman
Wilmington, NC

All rights reserved

ISBN-13: 978-1497559462
Printed in the United States of America

God also spoke to Moses and said to him: "I am the Lord. I appeared to

Abraham, Isaac, and Jacob as God Almighty, but by my name 'The Lord.' I did

not make myself known to them. I also established my covenant with them, to

give them the land of Canaan, the land in which they resided as aliens. I have

also heard the groaning of the Israelites whom the Egyptians are holding as

slaves, and I have remembered my covenant. Say therefore to the Israelites, 'I

am the Lord, and I will free you from the burdens of the Egyptians and deliver

you from slavery to them. I will redeem you with an outstretched arm and

with mighty acts of judgment.I will take you as my people, and I will be your

God. You shall know that I am the Lord your God, who has freed you from the

burdens of the Egyptians. I will bring you into the land that I swore to give to

Abraham, Isaac, and Jacob; I will give it to you for a possession. I am the Lord.'"

Exodus 6:2-8(NRSV)

My sincere and heartfelt gratitude for all those who diligently

labored along side me to make **Out of Obesity and into the**

Promised Land a reality. It was an honor to work with such

immensely gifted and extremely talented professionals—from

designers, artist, editors, and proofreaders, you are an integral

part of my success. Thank you, I could not have done it without

you. With your encouragement, expertise (and plenty of massage

sessions) we made it through to the end. I am especially proud to

include, among the best in their field, two of my own children.

Cover and Book Layout:
Brent Holloman - Brent Holloman Design

Before and After Photos:
Millie Holloman - Millie Holloman Photography

Editors:
Eileen Daigle
Charlene Dupray
Nancy Bolts
Jason Frye

Table of Contents

About the Author

Author Julia Holloman chose to undergo bariatric surgery in 2006, and won a life-long battle with her weight to lose 164 pounds. She now shares all that led to her remarkable success, including the wisdom she acquired, her quest for emotional and physical healing, and what was perhaps the most significant contributor of all: her extraordinary faith.

Since surgery Julia has become a certified bariatric coach with a critically acclaimed book, **Out of Obesity and into the Promised Land**. Her outreach also includes the leadership of a number of support and bible study groups, a blog (www.milestogoblog.com) that enjoys thousands of followers, and a public speaking tour.

A woman of immense Southern charm and purpose, Julia lives in Wilmington, North Carolina. She will be the first to tell you that her greatest gifts are her husband of 38 years, her children and grandchildren, and her relationship with God.

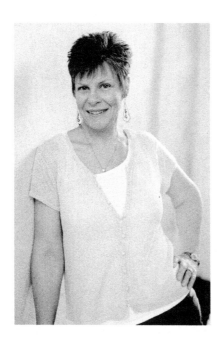

FORWARD

Out of Obesity and Into the Promised Land is Julia Holloman's personal story. But, I'd bet you a skinny sugar-free vanilla latte that much of her story is your story too! The land of obesity is no promised land. When it strikes, it is sure to leave its marks. Those marks are not just the physical.

Being human, we are all created with three dimensions; mind, body and spirit. Julia invites you to deal with all three. As healthcare providers, we tend to focus on the physical. This is unfortunate, because complete healing is never really achieved unless we deal with the mind, soul and spirit. This is never truer than when dealing with morbid obesity and weight loss surgery. A weight loss surgical procedure will never solve your obesity issue. You must be willing to do the mental and spiritual work to achieve lasting success. There is no other way. We cannot separate our body from the mind, soul, and spirit. It is imperative that you commit to the mental and spiritual care. Your insurance will require a psychological evaluation. Your surgeon will see to it that you meet that requirement. However, it is your responsibility to nurture your mind and your spirit. Operating on your stomach will not permanently change your mind. And denial will not make all of the issues that contribute to obesity go away. They are there and you must deal with them.

Julia compares her weight loss experience to the biblical journey of the Israelites as they made their way out of Egypt and into their Promised land. As a bariatric clinician, I have the joy of meeting and working with hundreds of weight loss patients each year. Just like the Israelites, these folks are ready for change. They have been beaten down and trodden by their disease. Weight loss surgery is their last hope. Often, they cannot see the Promised Land that awaits them. But, they are able to step out in faith because they know someone else made it. Yes! Just like the Israelites, faith will take them to a land that they never dreamed possible. And the same God that brought the Israelites to their land of plenty, their birthright and their destiny, will bring these weight loss surgery patients to their land of plenty. What they do when they get there is up to them.

I applaud Julia for caring enough to give us her story. It exposes her in a way that may not be comfortable. However, she is willing because she now lives in the promised land. It is not a perfect land, but it is a land full of promise. Julia did the hard work and she continues to do the hard work. Her journey is not over. Just like the Israelites, she will have to fight to remain in her promised land. And that is the point. Weight loss surgery is a lifetime commitment. It is a fight. But, it is a fight worth fighting. I urge you to put on all of your armor and prepare for battle. Julia is a warrior in the throes of the obesity fight. Join her!

Kim F. Joyner, *RN, CNOR*

New Hanover Regional Medical Center Bariatric Program Outcomes Manager
Vice President National Association of Bariatric Nurses (NABN)
Wilmington, North Carolina

We Never Walk Alone

With all my love to my husband Richard, my closest friend, faithful companion, constant support, tireless encourager, and intimate lover of more than 38 years, the first and only love of my life who loved me through thick and all the way to thin.

To our three most prized gifts in life, our three children, Seth, Millie, and Brent. You have blessed me beyond my wildest dreams. You hold within you everything you need to be all that you were created to be. Dream big, fly high, and always build your nest near the altar of His throne.

To our two divinely chosen and precious daughter-in-laws whom we now consider our own, Amanda and Dana. When you call me *Mom*, it's like music to my ears.

To four little ones who occupy a special place in our lives—the first little seedlings of the next generation—two little boys and two little girls who bear our family name and live entwined within our hearts, Gavin, Genevieve, Finn and Saylor. Life just doesn't get any better than grandchildren. MeMe's new lap was made ready for you and all who follow after.

You all have been my inspiration, motivation, and reason for reclaiming my health and pursuing all life has to offer. You all represent a forever promise that life will go on and I'm going with it. There are no words to express my love for you.

To my Daddy, (1928 – 1970) I miss him so much, but I'm still walking in his shadow.

To my Mother, the one who gave me the greatest of life's gifts: life and love. You raised two girls to adulthood by yourself. You and Daddy showed us what love looks like. You showed us how to live life after disappointment, through our greatest loss, how to be strong, how to pull through, how to choose happiness, and never give up—for this I am eternally grateful.

To my sister, Ginger, my parents' priceless and lifetime gift to me at the age of five. Always keep that beautiful smile and keep your head up. There are special treasures waiting for you one day.

To Papa Webb, I'm still "Little Weensy" on the inside; I just haven't always looked like it on the outside.

To my two faithful grandmothers, you planted in me seeds of faith and taught my heart to sing.

To Holly Ormond, my spiritual mother who introduced me to The Way, The Truth, and The Life. You directed me toward the good path, and offered a strong and firm foundation on which I could build the spiritual bridge in my life.

To the "Deborah Company" girls: Debbie, Lana, Sally, Vicki, and Vicky—you believed in me and encouraged me to follow the call of God on my life.

Among them are those who continued to stand closely by me gifting me with their love and support—physically, emotionally, and spiritually—including La Cretia and Jennifer.

To Anne and Udy, when I met you I had already been given my life back, but you helped to unwrap my "grave clothes." You have helped me receive more of God's grace and love, which satisfies my thirsty soul and fills my hungry heart.

I am thankful to all the professionals, being leaders in their field, in bariatrics and endocrinology for your excellent training and professional expertise: Dr. David R. Miles, bariatric surgeon and the staff at Miles Surgical, an ASMBS Bariatric Surgery Center of Excellence (BSCOE); Dr. Almond J. Drake III, MD, Endocrinology; and Dr. John C. Parker, MD, Endocrinology. I am grateful that I was given the opportunity to be under your watchful care, which offered me a way of escape and a return to improved health. I would like to add a special *thank you* to Dr. Miles to whom I dedicate this book (as well as my *Miles to Go blog*). Your professional care, commitment to excellence, and ongoing support have paved the road from impossible to possible and offered a new and healthier life for me as well as to many others, and allowed us to look forward to many more *miles to go*!

I am grateful for the nutritionists and dietitians, included among them are Heidi Kaufman MS, LDN, CDE, Clinical Nutritionist and Chaundra Klein Evans, RD, LDN, Nutrition Therapist who worked carefully and closely along side me. Your knowledge, time, and energy were crucial to my success.

I am thankful for those in the field of plastic surgery who had to work miracles just to make me fit inside my skin again: Dr. Al S. Aly, MD, FACS, and Dr. Albert E. Cram, MD, FACS of Iowa City Plastic Surgery. You did a terrific job.

To Miles Surgical Support Group Leader Kim Joyner, RN, CNOR, New Hanover Regional Medical Center Bariatric Program Outcomes Manager, I extend my gratitude for getting us headed in the right direction, leading us over the bumps in the road, setting us back on the right path when we stray, and cheering us on to the end.

I express my heartfelt gratitude for all those who have walked with me on the journey to freedom. These were the people who were the scaffolding and on whom I leaned for support and made it possible for me to build a strong foundation. They held me up when I couldn't hold up myself. This faithful support team has been a priceless gift. Among them were professionals, coaches, counselors, pastors, friends, and family who have offered me a helping hand, equipped me for the walk, lent a listening ear, encouraged me over obstacles, put me on the right path, and cheered me on to success.

I am ultimately thankful to The Lord. He went before me preparing the way. He has been my steady traveling guide and trusted companion. He has delivered me up out of the land of captivity, brought me into the land of promise and restoration, and enabled me to possess freedom in a new life. His love for me is unfathomable. Only in Him have I found that which is above all things, prosperity of soul, and the ultimate cure for my hungry heart—life eternal.

To all of you who read this book and the *Miles to Go blog*, and participants of Miles Surgical Bariatric Support Group, I celebrate with you, your new life, and I am delighted to be a part of your experience.

To all those who journey after, be encouraged along the way, and know that you are not alone, there are those of us who have gone before you and cleared the path. We, now, walk along side you, to cheer you on, and to ensure that the journey for you will be just a little easier. Success can be yours.

Yes, you can. Together, we will. We have many more *miles to go* as we walk out of obesity and into new and unexplored freedoms that await us in the Promised Land.

PART ONE:

The Road To Slavery

Life Before Surgery
A Slave in the Land of Obesity

Adversity is like a strong wind.
It tears away from us all but
the things that cannot be torn,
so that we see ourselves as
we really are.

Arthur Golden

The Turning Point

The lowest ebb is the turn of the tide.

Henry Wadsworth Longfellow

302.

There it was. The hard cold reality. It was both numbingly unbelievable and painfully certain.

The number that shook my world. It stared back at me, as the reality of the moment surrounded me like the cold metal bars of a prison. Life had suddenly moved from possibility to impossibility, from hope to hopelessness.

It was my fourth time on South Beach—not the white sandy shores dancing with golden rays of sunshine, painted sea shells, the smell of tropical suntan lotion, and yellow polka-dot bikinis—but the last desperate attempt on the road to weight loss. All my friends were on this newly discovered diet and losing weight like crazy, but not me. Just like the last three times, I had not lost one pound. Why had I hoped that this time would be any different?

As I stepped on the scale that day, I must have had a tiny fraction of hope that this time it would be different. Expecting to see even a small loss, a small ray of hope that somehow all the deprivation, all the donuts I had given up, and the French fries I had turned down, all the hours spent on that stationary bike going nowhere would account for something. As the bar sailed with a clang to the top of its little space, my heart sank. I stared in disbelief.

I had gained, again. Maybe it was only a few pounds, probably fluctuation. Maybe it was just too much salt the day before. But, whatever it was, moving that big bar over to the 300-pound space was a move that was beyond the boundary that held my hope in check. It was a move that changed my world—forever.

My weight had reached an all-time high of 302 pounds. I was in trouble. I had surpassed my ultimate limit—past the point I was willing to go. This last ditch effort had failed. Another diet, another disappointment, another failure. I needed help.

Out of Obesity by Julia Holloman

CHAPTER 1

Welcome to the Journey

Two roads diverged in a wood, and I, I took the one less traveled by, and that has made all the difference.

Robert Frost

It was at mile marker 302 that life's journey brought me to a fateful crossroad—one that held a life-changing decision to explore having Gastric Bypass Roux-en-Y (RNY) weight loss surgery. From that point on, my life was permanently influenced by the decision I made. It was the beginning of a new way of viewing life and planted me in a place of tremendous growth, even life anew.

This book chronicles my journey from obesity to improved health, from emotional bondage to personal freedom, and from years of struggle with "yo-yo" dieting to long-term weight loss success.

We all know that obesity is a huge issue, no pun intended. Eat less, exercise more, and you can lose all the weight you need and keep it off for life. I'm guessing that's not been your experience, either. Right?

After we have tried and failed all the ordinary methods, it seems that weight loss surgery is the answer, at least on the surface. Reduce the size of your stomach, eat less, and you're fixed for life. Now, you can live happily ever after. Well, it sounds good in theory. But is this reality?

Is undergoing bariatric surgery the right choice for you? The decision is certainly not an easy one. Weight loss surgery comes with risks as well as rewards. For most, this drastic measure is a last resort, a last chance, and the last hope on the weight loss road.

This means we need more than ever before to find success.

In reality, we know that diets don't work the magic they promise. Studies report that dieting offers a 95 percent failure rate. Even with our best effort, dieting only offers us about a 5 percent weight loss. Add in a little exercise and we might be able to push that percentage up to around 10 percent. Neither exercise nor diet pills have been proven effective in decreasing body fat or producing long-term weight loss for the morbidly obese. So, why do we think that smaller stomachs and smaller portions will be enough for the long haul? There has to be more.

Does weight loss surgery work? You bet. Having bariatric surgery offers a tool to help us lose weight and achieve a long-awaited dream of success. It gives those who need it a second chance. A chance to start over, make different choices, and attain improved health. A chance to find restoration, rebuild the future, and experience new opportunities.

For many, however, weight loss surgery has not been what they expected.

If you are considering weight loss surgery, I will tell you that it is not a "quick fix," an "easy way out" of obesity, or the "be all—end all" to life's problems. However, the good news is: you can find success. But what is success? What does it look like and what does it mean to you, personally?

Finding my way to success held far more than I ever imagined. My journey has led me to life altering and remarkable places that no diet could possibly take me.

For me, life after weight loss surgery has been more than an outward transformation. When my physical size started to decrease after surgery, I quickly realized that altering my physical anatomy wouldn't be enough to secure the transformation I was seeking. I found that it has required more than the physical adjustment to my anatomy, changes in diet, and a commitment to exercise in order to reach long-term weight loss.

Physically, I was prepared to confront surgery, but nothing prepared me for the emotional aspects of the journey or the long-term commitment it takes to keep the weight off.

After massive weight loss, my mind and body were not on the same page. I didn't recognize my reflection in the mirror. I knew all the tricks and rules for losing weight, but I knew very little about maintaining my success. I was winning the battle of the bulge, but I wasn't winning the battle of the mind. I discovered I needed to find health and success in other areas of my life, not just the physical.

It is here that I had to make my exit off the beaten path.

As a Christian, I love to read and study the Bible in-depth, but I had yet to find a Bible verse that outlined the best diet plan or how to control my insatiable desire for donuts and chocolate cake. After years of reading the Bible, I didn't realize the answers that would lead to my weight loss success were held within its pages. However, as I made my way out of obesity, I realized that there was a biblical story that seemed to closely parallel my own.

What follows are two stories: my struggle to escape obesity, and another—a biblical story. It is one of the oldest and greatest stories ever told. It is a story that spans the pages of the Old Testament and is deeply reflected in the New. It became a life-changing catalyst, unfolding inspiration and encouragement as I made my way into a healthier life—in body, mind, and spirit. It was this story of hope that providentially found its way into my life and miraculously continues to fill the empty corners of my heart. It was here that I found the missing keys that helped me to understand the source of my pain and set me free from the chains that held me in despair and discouragement.

I have discovered that shedding excess pounds on the outside offered me the prospect of improved physical health, but it was this inward passage that brought a release from heavy emotional weights and released me to experience new freedoms never before tasted.

I share my story because I believe that no matter where you are along your journey, you can enjoy the same success. It has become my passion to help others make their way to a healthier lifestyle, achieve lasting weight loss, and enjoy continued success after weight loss surgery.

No matter how unique we are, how differently our body reacts to surgery, or what circumstances we've encountered in life that have brought us here, we do have a few things in common. I have been where you are. I have known the frustration, hopelessness, and helplessness of being overtaken by the things that held me powerless to change. We have been walking the same path, we've been fighting the same battles, we have been hungry, wounded, and broken, and we have felt abandoned on the battlefield of life.

I found a way to escape from the grip of obesity. I want you to find it, too. You can start the journey on the right path, watch the weight fall off, return to physical, emotional, and spiritual health, discover the "new you" emerge with every step, and end victorious. I am here to walk with you to success, cheer you on to the finish line, help you discover life, and live it to the fullest.

If you are considering having weight loss surgery, this book will help you understand what lies ahead and how you can make the decisions that are right for you, prepare you for the passage, and help you reach and preserve personal success.

You may be a weight loss surgery patient just taking your first steps. If so, this book will help you make your way over obstacles and help clear the way to freedom that no diet has ever provided. My hope is that it will guide and encourage you.

This book is also for weight loss surgery patients who have completed the weight loss phase. You may be one, two, or more years out from surgery and now you are faced with keeping the weight off. You may be confused, frustrated, and disillusioned. Things aren't what you expected, and you need answers that allow you to reach your goal and maintain what you have worked so diligently to accomplish.

This book will also provide answers for those of you who may just have a few pounds to lose—maybe you're not considering weight loss surgery, but you have been repeatedly fighting the same losing battle. There will be healthcare differences in managing an altered anatomy after surgery, but the basic principles and lifestyle changes are the same. These principles will also help you find your way to success.

Although I may be speaking directly to those who are going through the weight loss surgery process, you may be a support person to a bariatric surgery patient or you may know someone who has had surgery or is seriously considering it. In this case, this book should serve to help you understand what is involved in weight loss surgery and aid you in supporting and encouraging others to achieve success—before, during, and after.

If you are considering weight loss surgery, it is important to find out everything you can about the types of bariatric surgeries, the different procedures that are available to you, and a qualified bariatric surgeon. Having realistic expectations of what these surgical treatments entail, discovering the meaning of personal success, educating yourself on the causes of obesity, and discovering the part you play in reaching your desired goal can mean the difference between *"Happily ever after"* and *"Houston, we have a problem."*

There are countless resources that detail the ever-changing physical, medical, and technical aspects of weight loss and surgery. This book is *not* a comprehensive resource on the causes of obesity. It does not offer a detailed guide of all weight loss surgery procedures. Nor, is it a substitute for medical advice. Rather it is a snapshot of my personal experiences and discoveries.

Are you tired of just *imagining* a life of freedom? Would you like to discover how to *live* there? Are you ready to uncover your true identity? Are you ready to discover your destiny, the one you were meant to fulfill? Are you ready for a lifetime of hunger to end? Isn't it time to lay aside the heavy weights you have been carrying for so long? Isn't it time to live your life? Isn't it time to experience new beginnings?

The road before us holds abundant hope and grace for each new day as we walk onward and upward into a brighter tomorrow. I invite you to come along, to share the transformations that changed my life—forever.

Buckle up! You're in for the adventure of a lifetime!

Having realistic expectations of what these surgical treatments entail, discovering the meaning of personal success, educating yourself on the causes of obesity, and discovering the part you play in reaching your desired goal can mean the difference between *"Happily ever after"* and *"Houston, we have a problem."*

Out of Obesity by Julia Holloman

CHAPTER 2

The Road to Here

Time is a dressmaker specializing in alterations.

Faith Baldwin

I grew up tall and thin. To my Grandpapa Webb—I was affectionately known as "Little Weensy." Although my parents never forced me to eat, or demanded I clean my plate, I can still recall my mother repeatedly telling me I was too little, and that I needed to eat—a statement she admitted regretting during my adult years. These statements usually followed our two annual shopping excursions into town for school clothes and her frustration to find clothing that fit me properly.

Our family was very close-knit, our extended family large, and our get-togethers frequent. Growing up near the family farms, food was always a part of what brought us together as a family all year round. Our summers were filled with planting vegetables in our backyard garden and canning produce. By the end of the summer, it was customary to find the entire clan gathered at the family home place, feasting on mounds of boiled peanuts and ice-cold bottled Pepsi-Cola and enjoying the playful company of my dad's six siblings and cousins beyond measure. Fall and winter brought the usual holidays, along with hog killings and going squirrel and rabbit hunting with my dad. We all looked forward to a visit from Aunt Frances and watching her make her prized peanut brittle. From milking cows to making memories, food was an integral and

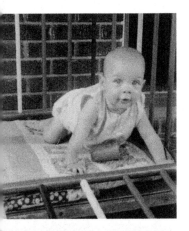

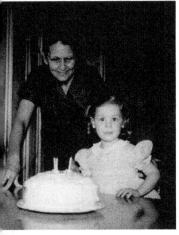

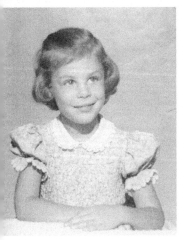

cherished part of my childhood years.

I remember being a good eater as a child. My food of choice—veggies. Among my favorites were anything green—collard greens, turnip greens, mustard greens, and butter beans. However, growing up in the south, (and eating at Papa and Mama Webb's house several times a week), I don't have to tell you that even the leafy greens were seasoned (along with generous amounts of love)—pork fat. Also from my mother's family table came traditions of fried cornbread and chicken with flour dumplings, known in the south as chicken pastry. My grandmother always thought that dessert should be eaten first. Fruit most often came in the form of jellies, jams, and homemade pies or turnovers filled with dried peaches or apples called "jacks"—which were, as you might guess, fried. My grandmother never thought it proper to leave her home without something edible in each hand. Such was life in a small farming community in eastern North Carolina in the 1950's and 60's.

Although, according to my childhood photos, I looked pretty normal. That was, until I met Richard. It was the summer of 1972. I was 15, preparing to enter the 10th grade. I still had that young, girlish figure, 120-125 pounds—small and slender on top, but complete with the family gift of a pear-shaped figure below. He was 18, ready to attend his first year of college. He was the proverbial tall, dark, and handsome and he won my heart pretty quickly. He was the first and only love of my life and we were married in 1975, just after I graduated from high school and he had completed college and secured a job.

Richard was an active athlete. He played any sport that included a ball—football, basketball, softball, golf, and tennis. Being raised on a family farm himself, he worked hard, ate whatever he wanted, whenever he wanted—without gaining an ounce. Whenever he ate, I did, too.

I entered marriage with a recipe box stuffed with recipes from pasta casseroles to homemade sweets. In those days, my idea of a good wife and southern cook was presenting a four-course dinner with all the trimmings, including biscuits and dessert. Richard didn't mind at all. I was a great cook. Add in a few rounds of birth control pills (which were changing me into someone I didn't like), plenty of time between business school classes to study and prepare great low-budget meals, and those first two years of marriage left me with a few extra pounds—25 pounds actually, and a new member of Weight Watchers.

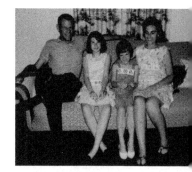

It worked—Weight Watchers and going off birth control. I lost 20 pounds. Back to my old self again. Just 5 more pounds to go, and I would accomplish my goal. But before I was able to lose those last 5 pounds, I became terribly ill. Something else had worked too. I just didn't know what it was, although I had my suspicions. I was either dying or I was pregnant. But weight loss was the farthest thing from my mind. It was survival time. I had a new job, we had a brand new home, and I had to feel better. I wasn't getting paid to hang around in the restroom all day. Saltine crackers and peanut butter became my staple foods. Soon, the test results confirmed the obvious—I wasn't dying, I was pregnant! We were so excited.

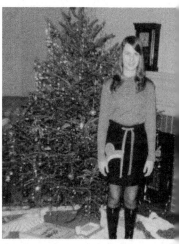

I ate to feel better so I could continue to work. By the time my first doctor's visit rolled around, the peanut butter crackers had recalled those 20 pounds.

The next few months brought on many changes, geographically as well as emotionally. It included a transfer in jobs for my husband and a move to another town. Each month, as my tummy grew, so did our excitement—along with my blood pressure and my weight. The pregnancy concluded with several weeks of bed rest, a salt-free diet, swollen feet, borderline toxemia (or preeclampsia), and a miserable 70-pound weight gain. The morning sickness turned into all-day sickness that followed me right into the labor and delivery room. By the end of the pregnancy, I weighed over 200 pounds.

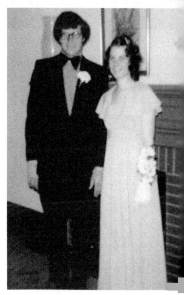

I did lose 30 pounds after giving birth to a beautiful 7-pound 12-ounce bouncing baby boy, which left me with 40 extra pounds to lose on my own. So, now on the agenda, along with being a first-time mom, was yet another diet.

I had no intention of remaining overweight. Over the next year or so, I tried several diets, but before reaching my goal—or

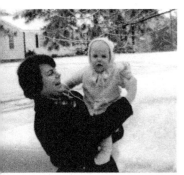

Seth (1979)

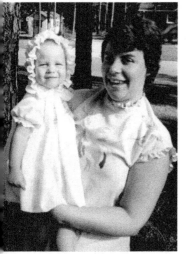

Millie (1981)

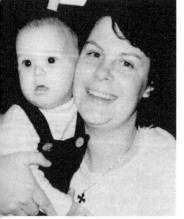

Brent (1983)

maintenance for that matter—I was pregnant with baby number two. This pregnancy was much smoother. I only gained a reasonable 25 pounds. You know what comes next in the cycle: have baby, lose weight, and then gain it back, plus a few. Eighteen months later, baby number three was on the way. Each time more dieting, each time returning to my former weight only to then surpass it and end up with more pounds than before I started.

Life was busy. I was happily married, and I loved being a fulltime wife and mother. But my life was also consumed with diets and losing weight. Slowly but surely it became a way of life.

Profession: Dieter

I became a diet professional. Weight Watchers, Overeaters Anonymous, Atkins, Nutri-Systems, LA Weight Loss, Medical Weight Loss, Professional Weight Loss, Sugar Busters, Jenny Craig, Slim Fast, Cardiac Nutritional Counseling, South Beach Diet, the Grapefruit Diet, the Cabbage Soup Diet, Weigh Down became "weigh up," and ended with "weigh" more of the same. If you sold it, I'd try it. There must have been hundreds. No caffeine, no soft drinks, no fat, no white sugar. Low sugar, low salt, more fiber, more failure, more frustration, more weight gain, and the only thing fried was me!

I spent twelve weeks with a nutritional counselor at the Cardiac Unit of our local medical center. She was so proud of my efforts. Each week I would come with my food journal, and we would talk about what I had eaten. The food was so tasteless I wondered why I was eating anyway. Sadly, week after week there was no weight loss. *"You're doing so well,"* she would say as she cheered me on. Inside, I was dying. *"Really? I came to lose weight. If I'm doing so well, why isn't the scale moving?"* I remember sitting in the car after each visit and crying as if my heart were broken. Didn't anyone understand that I was really trying? That I wasn't eating to look like that. I might have eaten like that before and I admitted to having made wrong choices in the past. But I was changing the way I ate. I was walking miles everyday, rain or shine, and I was not cheating—no donuts, no cake, no soda, no fat, and certainly no chocolate. I had to give up chocolate years before in order to control my migraine headaches. Do you know how few candy bars there are that don't contain chocolate? Not many! And by all means, let's not forget the Tums I ate. Did I have to record those on my diet sheet?

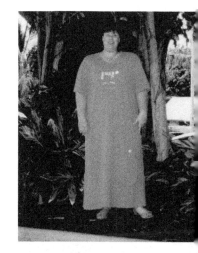

I had tried so many diets, gained and lost so many times that, over the years, my body started to rebel. Diets were just not working anymore. That's when I started to consult with doctors about my thyroid, estrogen dominance, yeast overgrowth, Wilson's disease, and Cushing disease. I was convinced there had to be something physically wrong with me.

As the years rolled by, it was more of the same: more diets, more doctors, more exercise programs, more tasteless food, more deprivation, and more weight gain. Then some new issues were added: high blood pressure, pre-diabetes, thyroid nodules, high cholesterol, high triglycerides, knee problems, joint pain, and sleep apnea.

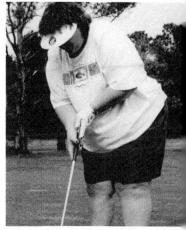

With a strong family history on both sides of heart disease and diabetes, I was beginning to be concerned. Not to mention the dashed dream of being "thin before thirty" or even forty, for that matter. Then around my 45th birthday, several of my first cousins died of heart attacks, with little or no warning. I began to worry. All five of my dad's brothers had heart disease, and most died prematurely. My grandmother and several of my mother's sisters had diabetes. One of the girls died at age 27 after going into a diabetic coma. My dad passed away at age 41 having suffered with high blood pressure, a debilitating stroke, and then finally a sudden fatal heart attack.

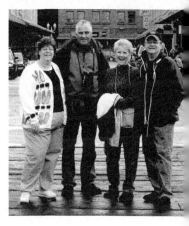

I did have a few successful weight loss experiences here and there. I had managed to lose 50 pounds by cutting calories and counting carbs (a plan I put together myself), and was desperately trying to keep it off. When I mentioned my efforts to my doctor and how hard I was trying just to hold on to the weight loss, his comment was that since I was getting older, I would just have to try harder. So I did.

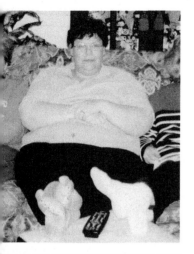

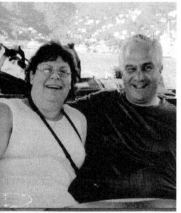

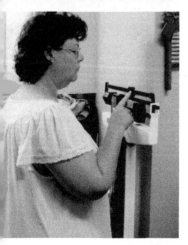

It was during this time that I decided to join LA Weight Loss, because a friend had experienced great results. As I watched her get smaller and smaller, I decided to give it a try. By the time I joined and bought the special bars and other foods, I had spent about $1,000.

I did lose—10 pounds the first two weeks. Wow, amazing! Then 5. Then it happened. What I had dreaded all along. I gained 10 pounds while still on the program. As usual, I would bring in my little diet journal, and they would tell me how well I was doing and that I would start losing again soon. Sometime later, I discovered that the cholesterol medications I was taking were adding to my weight gain. They were also making me terribly sick.

After much experimentation, I ended my last round of cholesterol medication with severe bladder spasms. Now unable to take any of those medications, I began to worry that I would be next in line for heart problems. People in my family weren't getting second chances, so I decided to get a check-up with a cardiologist. To my utter amazement, my blood pressure was extremely high. I was devastated. It took months of trial and error and many combinations of drugs to bring it somewhat under control.

Over the years, I had seen a number of doctors who offered varied advice from eating only half of a sandwich instead of a whole one to having weight loss surgery. A half of a sandwich? Are you kidding me? This was far more than just eating a half of a sandwich. Wasn't anyone listening to my cry for help? I needed real answers. I had a real problem. Diets were not helping me; I had tried and retried them all. But, weight loss surgery—out of the question. Not me. No one was going to change MY anatomy. That was certainly not the answer. I had known too many people who had undergone weight loss surgery only to find themselves right back where they started.

Ultimately, I had determined that something had to be wrong with my body. But the only advice doctors offered left me feeling as if I had not tried hard enough or that I was in denial. Instead of being faithful to the diet, maybe I was "cheating." I felt as though my integrity was in question. *"Are you bingeing?"* some would ask. I had begun to doubt my ability to be honest with myself. I felt as though people judged me as weak, lazy, undisciplined, and without self-control—and now, dishonest. Did they think I really wanted to be like that, or that maybe I hadn't noticed that I was wearing a 3X? Or maybe they thought I was happy with the way things were.

As my weight continued to climb, Richard's patience was wearing thin. I was desperate for an answer.

An endocrinologist who I was seeing for my thyroid had recommended another diet, and this, just after his long spiel on burning more calories than I took in. *"A diet? Why, I never thought of that!"*

He recommended the South Beach Diet (which I had already tried three times without success) in combination with hiring a personal trainer. Just like the last gazillion efforts, the scale didn't budge an inch. Well, actually, that's not true. It did move, but not in the losing direction.

Out of Obesity by Julia Holloman

CHAPTER 3

In Search of the Promised Land

But I have said to you, 'You shall inherit their land, and I will give it to you to possess, a land flowing with milk and honey.'
Leviticus 20:24 (ESV)

It seemed all my efforts to work harder, eat less, and exercise more, were leading me further and further away from my intention. But even in the midst of the struggle to lose weight, I was also struggling to hold on to a promise.

In 1995, just before we moved our family from Greenville, NC, a few hours south to Wilmington, NC, I found a story in the bible that captured my attention. It was in the book of *Exodus* (23:20-33).

In this story, the Israelites had been delivered out of slavery and were waiting to go into their Promised Land. As they wait to make their transition into a new place, God promises to send an angel ahead of them to prepare the way, guard them, and lead them to their destination. At the time, this passage really helped me make the transition of moving to a new place in my life geographically. But as time went on, these verses began to hold even greater significance.

The *Exodus* story actually begins in the book of *Genesis*, with a man named Abram. Abram was chosen by God and given a promise of a new life. God had promised to make him the father of many nations, yet he and his wife, Sara, remained childless. He promised him and his children a place of rest and restoration—a land of inheritance, where they could live their lives in peace and fulfillment. God also changed Abram's name to Abraham, and his wife's name to Sarah, as a reminder of His promise. Abraham held within him the seeds and the faith to see the promise fulfilled, even though on the outside there was no indications at all that it would happen.

God did fulfill His promise to Abraham and Sarah. In their old age, well beyond their childbearing years, they had a son named Isaac. Isaac had a son named Jacob, whose name was changed to Israel. Later, in a bizarre turn of events, one of Israel's sons, Joseph, was forsaken by his brothers and sold into slavery in the land of Egypt. Falsely accused, Joseph was thrown into prison and forgotten. As time passed, Joseph was eventually restored and given a place of authority.

Seeking refuge from a famine, the entire family was instructed by God to move to Egypt, where Joseph had been strategically placed in a position to save his family from starvation.

Over the course of time, this small family (known as the Israelites) grew in number. They arrived as honored guests, but soon they became a threat to the Pharaoh, and found themselves suffering immense cruelty. Eventually they became enslaved in a life of intense labor. They were commanded to build cities, labor in the fields, and make bricks. As time went on, they were demanded to perform their brickmaking task with no provisions by which to accomplish it. They felt as if no one was listening to their cries for help—and once again the promise of dwelling in the land of freedom seemed impossible.

Through it all, God had promised them that He would be with them, that they would become a great nation, and little by little, they would possess the land.

He was faithful to His promise. He responded to their cries for help and sent a liberator to rescue them up out of the land of slavery.

Just like Abraham, I was holding tightly to some promises of my own. I had begun to pray for my own Promised Land. Someday, surely I would reach the place for which I longed—a land that offered me an escape from the physical bondage of obesity and offered a much needed rest from my never ending battle to lose weight.

Many times, I read the story. I stood with Abraham on a hillside as God showed him the land of promise. Daily I studied the scriptures of how God delivered his descendants from their oppression at the hands of an unmerciful ruler. I began to study their journey as they were released from slavery in Egypt and made their way through the Red Sea.

For years I studied the details of their journey from the book of *Genesis* through the book of *Joshua*. I followed the generations as they made their way across the wilderness and battled their way through seemingly impossible circumstances until little by little they conquered their enemies, discovered their true identity, and came to possess the land of their dreams.

I, too, had heard the sounds of faith. They drew me onward and exhorted me to be strong and courageous—to go in and take possession of my Promised Land.

For years, I held fast to promises of breaking free from the oppression and despair, in hopes that restoration would come and I could rebuild a life in health. Each day, I searched for answers, made attempts at wiser food choices, struggled to remain compliant to my diet and exercise plan—and with it I rehearsed the promises of living life in a new place of freedom. But outwardly, there was no sign of change and my freedom also seemed questionable.

Whispers in the Night

Although I didn't realize it at the time, I was being prepared for the change that would come. As I look back, I can see the change had started even then—changes on the inside were taking place long before I ever thought about having weight loss surgery.

I recall one day in particular. Among other transitions going on in my life at the time, I was on yet another quest to lose weight. Imagine that.

It was February 14, 2001. It was in a pretty dark season in my life and everything within me had been resounding with loud cries for help. The weather that particular day was dreary, cold, and rainy. I picked up a well-worn devotional book and read the scripture for the day. The entry, *Matthew 10:37 (KJV): "What I tell you in the dark, speak in the light; what is whispered in your ear, proclaim from the roofs."* My hopeless cries needed to be quieted so that I could hear.

What was there to hear? Whispers? Were there whispers? Sounds of hope? Anywhere? Really?

I remember going to a prayer group that morning. My seat was diagonally across from a sliding glass door. Sitting there, still, the prayers in the room seemed to fade into the background. The dreariness outside called my attention to the stark and lifeless face of the winter scene. Trees with no leaves—snarled and bent—identifiably, cold and lifeless.

Thoughts like whispers came. Taking center stage was a still, quiet, familiar voice from within. *"Listen."*

I knew enough science to know that the trees were not dead. For hidden in the dark, buried deep in the soil there were roots preparing for spring. Although it's true that tree roots grow more fervently during warmer months, there was life and growth nevertheless.

A term that more aptly describes root growth in the winter is referred to as *"resting but ready."* This readiness is extremely important for the individual health of each tree and, therefore, ensures the health and well-being of the whole forest.

This is extremely important, this trait of readiness, for it allows trees to absorb water and avoid winter dehydration. This is the time when trees are given the opportunity to expand their root systems in search of water and nutrients in advance of spring and to prepare for what is to come. They have work to do, a purpose to fulfill. They also know something that is not obvious above ground: life and spring are approaching soon, for new life is a sure and coming promise, waiting.

I really couldn't shake that image or the verse running through my head that day. I felt the need to surrender. It was like the picture of the tree. In order for the new leaves of spring to come, the green leaves of summer need to surrender to the vibrant colors of the fall, and then to the call of winter. To us, it looks like the end; but it is really a picture of renewal. For if there is no letting go of the past, there will be no hope for the new to appear.

And so, that night, at the end of a pew, in a small little church, with my face to the floor, I surrendered to God all my hopes and plans. I certainly hadn't been able to change things myself. Maybe He would.

During this dark season, I became still enough to listen. There were things I needed to hear and learn in that dark place. For darkness doesn't mean lifelessness. Like those trees, God was preparing me for change to come. During those next few years, even though things with my weight didn't appear to be changing, He, all the while was making me ready on the inside. He was whispering things I would need to hear in order to bring me to a place of renewal.

At the time, I was growing spiritually and in faith by leaps and bounds; but, outwardly, there was nothing to see. I was listening and it was my season of "resting but ready." I'm not so sure how well I was resting, but I was extremely ready for change to come. Nevertheless, I made listening my focus.

As time passed, matters seemed to get worse. With each repeated attempt and weight loss failure, my hope of freedom was sinking in a sea of despair. With one hand I held on to the promise of restoration and with the other I found myself grasping hold of discouragement and hopelessness—believing that things were never going to be any different and that I would forever remain overweight, unhealthy, and unchanged.

So here I was: December 2005, South Beach Diet for the fourth time with a personal trainer to boot. This one last hope and futile effort to change things had ended in disaster, and moving that bar from 299 to 302 was the tipping point. With the move of that bar, my world had suddenly turned upside down. It seemed as though I was struggling to overcome the impossible. I was imprisoned in a body I hated, and it was devouring my life. There seemed to be no way out.

CHAPTER 4

Casual Corners Become
Divine Intersections

There is no medicine like hope, no incentive so great, and no tonic so powerful as expectation of something tomorrow.

Orison Swett Marden

For the Israelites, it must have seemed there was no way out, as well. In the land of Egypt, the Pharaoh had instituted a law that every baby boy born to the Hebrews must be thrown into the river Nile. But even in the worst of times, God had a Master Plan. There was still a thread of hope that remained alive and God had already prepared a way of escape.

One little baby boy had been spared; his name was Moses. Rescued by the Pharaoh's daughter, he was given a special education and favored position in the land. It appeared he was the answer they had been looking for. But when Moses comes to the aid of a fellow Hebrew, things went fatally wrong and he fled Egypt to live his life in the desert and with him their hope of being rescued disappeared once again.

All the while God had a special plan and purpose for Moses. He was being prepared to deliver God's chosen people out of slavery and into the Promised Land. Suddenly one day, forty years later, Moses was commissioned by God to lead the Hebrews out of Egypt. So Moses returned to Egypt to free the captives and restore their hope.

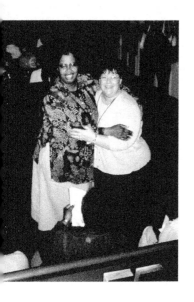

It was at that moment that I realized that Casual Corner had become a divine intersection.

Life is like that. Sometimes, when you least expect it, things can take a sudden turn.

In the fall of 2003, three of my close friends joined me in purchasing tickets for a live filming of a Bible study series led by Beth Moore, a well-known Christian author and public speaker. As the date drew closer, two of the girls had to cancel. Nevertheless, my friend Melissa and I set out for the long drive to Baltimore, Maryland. It proved to be a harrowing trip through pouring rain and heavy fog. Even though driving in such conditions on unfamiliar roads was my worst nightmare, I felt compelled to continue on.

When we arrived in Baltimore, I told Melissa that I wanted to stop at Casual Corner to look at clothing for an upcoming event. As we shopped in the store, the sales associate asked, *"Are you here to see Beth Moore?"* What were the chances that, in a large city, our sales associate would actually know of Beth Moore? She went on to tell us that her entire Bible study group was going to the event, but she had not been able to purchase a ticket.

"The session begins in a few hours, if you had a ticket, would you be able to make it?" I asked. *"Yes, I could go,"* she replied. As I proceeded to pay for my purchase, I handed her one of the unused tickets. When she saw the ticket, tears filled her eyes. *"You're giving me a ticket?"* she asked. As we hugged, cried, and rejoiced across the checkout counter, she relayed her story: *"I have been praying for a way to attend this event. All of my friends have been making plans to attend, but funds have been tight and there was no way I could afford a $70 ticket. I felt like God had completely forgotten me, or that He hadn't heard my prayers."*

"What is your name?" I asked. *"Dee Evans,"* she replied. It was at that moment that I realized that Casual Corner had become a divine intersection. *"Dee, God has not forgotten you, He heard your prayer. This ticket has been reserved with your name on it for the past nine months. My friend who purchased this ticket had to cancel at the last minute—her name is also Dee Evans."*

We marveled at God's timing. He had been way ahead of her, preparing and orchestrating each and every detail. What an amazing privilege to be used to bring a demonstration of hope and answered prayer to someone waiting.

In the same way, I was deep in the throes of my struggle with obesity and I needed a deliverer as well. Little did I know that God had already laid the groundwork. He had heard my cries for help and He had already prepared the answer years before I would need it. And even though I couldn't see it at the time, He would be faithful to His promise.

My answer would take the form of a childhood classmate. Al Drake and I were in the same grade at South Edgecombe School from elementary through high school. After high school, we went our separate ways. While I got married and started a family, he went to medical school. It was no surprise to me—he was always at the top of the class. In 2005, an extended member of my family told me that Al was now Dr. Al Drake, Chief Endocrinologist at the East Carolina School of Medicine in Greenville, NC. Desperate to find a solution, I decided that my friend, Al, might be able to give me the answer that I was seeking. I knew his character was one of honesty, and I trusted that he would give his medical opinion with excellent professional expertise and sincere personal concern. It would be my last and final hope. If he didn't have a solution, I would give up and just forget the whole diet thing altogether. I would admit defeat once and for all.

So, on December 28, 2005, I made the 2-hour trip to meet with him.

The Visit with the Doctor

Was I prepared for another disappointment?

Other professionals had spent their time informing me about the "ins and outs" of caloric intake, explaining that I had to eat less and exercise more. It was like telling me to make bricks with no straw. *"Make more bricks, make more bricks. Try harder. No, harder. Are you lazy?"* But the harder I worked, the more hopeless I felt.

Would Dr. Drake hear my cries for help? Would I find the answers I needed?

Dr. Drake listened as I expressed my frustration in trying to lose weight without success. Listening gave me validation. He validated my efforts on having done the best that I could. That was at least a start. No one else had given me any credit at all for all the years of effort I had put into losing weight. I so desperately needed to know that, finally, someone believed I was really sincere.

He explained that my weight was like trying to hold down a large spring. It takes effort to hold it down, but when you lighten up on the pressure, or take your hand off, it flies out of control. That was exactly how I felt. It was a great visual. Finally there was someone who could relate to my dilemma.

He conveyed that the problem was not that I hadn't tried, but that there were things limiting my efforts that I had not known. He suggested many possible causes of obesity including genetics, hormonal imbalances, medications, and environmental related issues.

Most of these causes I had heard or read about before. But he did mention a few things I had never considered. One was my liver. I learned that the liver (one of the largest and most important organs in the body) can be adversely affected by morbid obesity. The liver has more than 600 functions, several of which are vital for weight control. That is, if it isn't impaired.

What could cause our liver to be impaired? One of the reasons is an accumulation of fat called *steatosis*. The risks associated with steatosis include diabetes, protein malnutrition, hypertension, and obesity. A fatty liver was perhaps hindering me from losing weight.

We also discussed the effects of "yo-yo" dieting and the detrimental effect of repeated up-and-down fluctuations of weight on the body's rate of metabolism, which results in the inability to lose weight effectively. He explained that since my body was over 100 pounds overweight, it was almost impossible for me to lose adequate weight on my own. Years of dieting had taken its toll. Not only had it defeated me emotionally, but it had made my body essentially more resistant to diet-induced weight loss. My body was now working against me. There was certainly a medical reason behind my failure, at least to some degree. Why hadn't someone explained this to me before?

Dr. Drake did suggest weight loss surgery as a possible solution. For the first time, I discovered that it wasn't a *fix* to the problem but instead, a *tool* that would offer me the jumpstart I needed.

I felt mixed emotions. It was frustrating to learn that discipline and hard work were sometimes not enough, and that there were actual biological forces working against me.

It was also a relief. After so many years of dieting with no success, and so many professionals questioning my efforts and ability to stick to diets, I had begun to doubt my ability to be faithful, diligent, and honest with myself. To be heard by Dr. Drake and to finally have a professional acknowledge that I had made an honest effort restored my self-confidence. I didn't realize the full impact of his validation at the time, but I now recognize that this is where my healing began.

Armed not only with the necessary medical information, but also with the permission to believe in myself, I now had a better understanding of how my body worked, how weight–loss surgery worked, and how it could aid me in losing weight.

Don't get me wrong; I'm not blaming my obesity on my liver. I take full responsibility for the poor eating habits, unwise choices, and yo-yo dieting that had gotten me there in the first place.

Was weight loss surgery my answer? I couldn't believe I was actually looking at it as a possibility. It was against everything I considered realistic or natural. Was it possible I had just been handed a small piece of hope? If the gift of weight loss I had longed for was packaged as weight loss surgery, I certainty didn't like the wrapping.

I do remember the walk to the car. I was in a daze—caught up somewhere between a slow motion echo of disbelief and the fast pace convergence of reality. Like any place of convergence, the waters were rougher than I expected. I wasn't sure if I had just been thrown a life raft or if I was being thrown overboard.

I soon realized that I had found what I had come for—hope. *Hope* is defined as "a feeling that what is desired is also possible." After all, if I still had any remnant of hope remaining, this might be the place to put it to work.

My hope may have been small, but what little I did have was beginning to be revived. Was it enough to awaken my dream? Was it enough to make it happen?

That day as I made my way from the lobby of the medical building, and turned the corner to Dr. Drake's office, I had no idea that this "casual corner" would become *my* divine intersection. My endless struggle to accomplish the impossible was about to come to a screeching halt. This turn marked the end of a road filled with diets, failure, and defeat, and it marked the beginning of a new road of hope and freedom—a new beginning, a new life, and a new destiny.

It was also no coincidence that my riding companion that day was my friend, Lana. Lana was also placed in my life under divine direction—like an angel who goes before you, softly speaking truth and good news. Lana reminded me of my dream and of God's promise. She would tell me over and over, *"God is preparing you for something that He has already prepared for you."* It was good to remember that someone had a plan, even if I didn't know where the road would lead, it renewed my hope that the Promised Land I longed for, was out there somewhere, waiting.

PART TWO:

Preparing For Departure

Weight Loss Surgery Phase One:
The Pre-Surgical Physical and
Emotional Preparation

**You can never cross the ocean
until you have the courage to
lose sight of the shore.**
Christopher Columbus

Dreams, Fears, Faith, and Decisions

**Faith is taking the first step even
when you don't see the whole staircase.**

Martin Luther King, Jr.

Somewhere between Diet 65 and Diet 965, I had laid aside my dream of ever being normal again. With my hope restored, there was plenty to consider. What did I want? What were my goals? Did I want to take the path of weight loss surgery? Would the end result be worth the physical and emotional price I would pay? It was time to go back for the dreams I had laid down so long ago, dust them off, and embrace them once again.

More than anything, I wanted to be normal, whatever normal meant. I wanted to go shopping for clothes in a regular clothing store, even if that meant Target or Wal-Mart. They might carry 3X size clothing, but they didn't fit me. I usually found that larger size clothing was poorly constructed, and made me feel old and frumpy. I was frustrated with expensive options. I wanted to, at least, be able to *try on* clothes at Ann Taylor.

I wanted to be able to sit in a plastic lawn chair without fear of breaking it. I wanted to go to a restaurant, sit in a booth, and still be able to eat. Most of time the food that was intended for my mouth ended up on my clothing in the process. I wanted to be able to pick up items I dropped on the floor and not wonder if I could retrieve them. I wanted to sit in a chair and cross my legs. I wanted to be able to fly in a plane without the embarrassment of having to ask for a seatbelt extension. I wanted to be able to run and play with grandchildren. I wanted to live again. I wanted a life.

I wanted to be healthy. I did not want to develop full-blown diabetes, have a stroke, suffer from heart disease, endure a debilitating illness, or die a premature death. I wanted to be off all prescription drugs and avoid all the side effects of artificial medication. I wanted my life back.

That was just the physical. I wanted to go to social events without feeling ostracized, depressed, embarrassed, and insignificant. I also wanted peace and joy. I wanted to like myself. I wanted to trust myself and to believe in myself. I wanted to be free from who I was on the inside. I wanted to be and feel attractive—especially to my husband. I wanted to feel good about who I was. I wanted self-control.

For so many years I had held on to the promise that life could be different and that out there somewhere was the promise of better health and emotional freedom. Even though the vision of possessing the land of promise was fading with each passing failure, I wanted to believe it could still happen. I wanted to hope again. I wanted to be free from defeat and hopelessness. I longed to be free from the oppression of an emotional prison. I wanted freedom.

CHAPTER 5

Crossover Considerations

It is part of the cure to want to be cured.
Roman Philosopher Lucius Seneca

As I began to consider weight loss surgery as an option, I had no idea that I had officially entered the first of four weight loss surgery phases. There are four general phases of weight loss surgery recognized by medical professionals.

These four phases include:

1. **The Pre-Surgical Phase**
2. **The Post-Surgical Physical Adjustment Phase**
3. **The Post-Surgical Psychosocial Adjustment Phase**
4. **The Long-term Maintenance Phase**

Phase One
The Pre-Surgical Phase—Preparations for Surgery

This first phase is the Pre-Surgical Phase, referred to as "pre-op." It is a time for gathering information and making decisions. This process includes discovering what weight loss surgery entails, learning about the available procedures, deciding whether weight loss surgery is the right choice, and preparing for life after surgery.

Deciding whether to have surgery is not an easy decision. We are about to be bombarded with information and there are lots of things to consider and questions that need answers. Life ahead seems very uncertain.

Q   Where do we start?

Q   How do we make the right decision?

I'm so glad you asked. For me, it began just as it did with the children of Israel as they were making their departure out of Egypt and preparing to enter into a new land.

Remember, God had called upon Moses to rescue the people from slavery in Egypt. This was an opportunity for Moses to fulfill his purpose in life. This opportunity came with great responsibility, and the responsibility came with a huge risk. He couldn't just walk in from the desert after 40 years and announce, *"Grab your bags, we're out of here!"* In order to lead them out, he had to risk standing before the Pharaoh.

Moses faced the fear of failure. He didn't see himself as a speaker. Actually it was quite the opposite. He had a speech impediment. Nevertheless, he would have to convince the Pharaoh to let the people go. This would require a huge step of faith on the part of Moses, and for the Israelites, too.

The Israelites had been enslaved in the land of Egypt for years. The only certainty they had was the promise that there was a land out there somewhere—a seemingly distant homeland, only as visible as the stories of those who once recalled it. They have heard that the land was rich and fertile—offering them freedom from slavery. But, slavery was all they knew. They had no idea what lay beyond the boundaries of their present life.

For although their destination was not far away, Moses knew what lay between them and their Promised Land. He knew the way was not easy, the terrain unfamiliar, the battles imminent, and their arrival time uncertain.

Just like any trip, the people needed to be prepared for the exodus out of Egypt. This would require informing them about the plan of escape and making necessary preparations for their departure. Once out of Egypt, they would need to be equipped to make the difficult journey across a desert and instructed on how to avoid trouble along the way. They would also need to be prepared for rebuilding a new life in a new place.

As we make our journey out of obesity and into a new land, we will also find it important to be informed, prepared, and equipped. These are important stepping-stones in this pre-surgery process. They will serve to ensure that we make an informed decision, position us for a more timely surgery date, provide us with a smoother journey, equip us for the challenges ahead, and allow us a successful transition into our new way of life.

This pre-surgical phase will include:

Gathering Information and Making Decisions

We need information. Knowledge helps us face our fears of the unknown and assists us in making informed decisions.

Physical Preparations

The pre-surgery phase will include preparations to make certain we are *physically* ready to move on to surgery. It will be important to find out everything we can about bariatric surgery, the different procedures that are available to us, and a qualified bariatric surgeon. We will need instructions for a safe surgery and information about how to make the transition into a new way of life.

Emotional Readiness

Knowing what surgery includes is one thing, but there are things to be considered beyond making the decision to have surgery. We must discover if we are mentally and emotionally ready for surgery. Emotional preparedness can help us calm our inward turmoil. Most weight loss patients will agree, we may be prepared *physically* for surgery, but few of us are *emotionally* prepared for the journey.

> As we make our journey out of obesity and into a new land, we will also find it important to be informed, prepared, and equipped.

I believe our emotional readiness is perhaps the most important part of the process. Pre-surgical emotional preparedness, as well as the understanding and making of post-surgical emotional adjustments, will be foundationally imperative to our long-term success. After years of being overweight, I was discouraged. I needed to believe that I could accomplish the task.

Arming for battle

Preparing for departure includes "leaving Egypt" and acknowledging the need to let go of the old way of life.

The way ahead will not be easy or fast. We must arm ourselves for rough terrain and the battles along our path. Life will present many challenges as we transition through each stage from pre-surgery, through massive weight loss, and into maintenance. This process will include the need for gathering fellow travelers and making plans for the journey. We will also need to arm ourselves with accurate expectations of what we can expect life to be like once we reach our Promised Land.

Equipping to rebuild

The Hebrews left with clothing, gold, and silver—supplies and materials they would need to rebuild their life in a new place. For me, making sure I was equipped for life in a new place proved just as valuable.

As you can see, there is more to this process than just finding out about the surgery itself—far more. Knowing these stages exist and how to maneuver through them is like having an on-board GPS—assisting you though the journey and helping you to finish victoriously.

As we begin to look at this pre-surgery phase and what it entails, I'll give you a few tips on how you can maneuver through this bewildering desert of decision and use this time to get ready for all that lies ahead.

Your weight loss surgery journey may not follow my exact path, but we will all pass certain mile-markers along the way.

CHAPTER 6

Happy Feet and Simple Steps

Great is the art of beginning, but greater is the art of ending.
Henry Wadsworth Longfellow

We'll start our decision making process with simple steps and a few questions. Oh, yeah, just what you need, more questions. These questions, however, are not just *about* surgery (we'll get to that). For now, there are questions you need to ask about *yourself*. Unlike the questions you have *about* surgery, I'm confident you have the answers to these. Let's go retrieve them.

Like most journeys in life, it starts with one step at a time. Simple steps will lead us in the direction of our choice.

The first question is; *What choice do we want to make?* Our heart will ultimately lead us in the direction we deem important. So it will be important to find out what is important, where our values lie, and what direction will take us to our anticipated destiny.

Taking inventory, creating a list, and counting the cost are essential components for any successful venture. Whether we are baking a cake, going grocery shopping, packing for a trip, or making life-changing decisions such as weight loss surgery—taking stock of our personal inventory, identifying where we are, and knowing where we're headed will equip us for success and silence the fears of uncertainty.

We can begin by writing down our thoughts. Writing brings clarity and helps us move forward. So grab a paper and pencil and begin by asking yourself questions, collecting your thoughts, and making lists.

No matter where you are in your journey—whether you have already made your decision to have surgery, or have already undergone surgery, I believe these steps are very important.

We can conquer those overwhelming moments by reconnecting with the present.

Q What does my life look like right now?

Q Is the path I am on giving me the results I desire?

The place where you find yourself right now is just a season. The great thing about seasons is that they change pretty quickly.

Stop and think about where you were 3 years ago, or what was happening in your life 5 years ago, or 10 years ago. Things in your life are probably much different than they were then. You have moved on to a new season. During the next few months and years, you will again move on to a whole new set of circumstances. Things do change. From here, it's important to think about where you are in the process and what you want the next few years of your life to look like.

Q Am I ready to move on to another season in my life?

Q What *do I know* already that can help me make this decision?

Q What things can I learn in this place where I am right now?

Q What can I do?

Q What present task do I need to complete?

...the reasons you choose to have surgery will have a direct impact on your success.

Although my purpose is not to tell you whether you should have surgery or not, I will tell you that the reasons you choose to have surgery will have a direct impact on your success. If your goals are to improve or return to health or find personal success for the long-term, it will serve to keep you focused for the long-term. I can tell you, as a word of caution, if the primary reasons you want surgery are based on temporary motivators—however beneficial, important, honorable, sincere, or totally legitimate—when your objectives are reached, you may experience short-term results.

Weight loss surgery is a drastic, life-changing measure, which carries tremendous risk and requires great diligence. This decision is a matter of life and death; and it should be taken seriously. Surgery is designed to give you weight loss success for a lifetime. Be sure your primary motivation for surgery will take you into long-term success.

It will be helpful to make a list of what you want to accomplish and what you expect the surgery to provide. This step will be helpful in determining whether your expectations are realistic and whether you are ready to move forward.

As I mentioned earlier, even if you have already had surgery, writing down the reasons why you had surgery will be a tremendous advantage for the long-term.

- **Q** What do I really want?
- **Q** What do I hope to accomplish?
- **Q** Why do I need or want surgery?
- **Q** What things do I want or need to change?
- **Q** What do I value?
- **Q** What do I want success to look like for me personally?
- **Q** What is success worth to me?
- **Q** Am I willing to pay the price it demands?
- **Q** What benefits will there be in losing weight?
- **Q** What do I expect the surgery to deliver?
- **Q** What things are holding me back?
- **Q** Will this step be a proper and suitable fit for my life, values, and personality?
- **Q** Who could I be right now?
- **Q** What do I expect the outcome of surgery to include?
- **Q** Do I have a realistic expectation of the outcome surgery offers?
- **Q** What additional available information do I need to know before moving forward?

> It will be helpful to make a list of what you want to accomplish and what you expect the surgery to provide. This step will be helpful in determining whether your expectations are realistic and whether you are ready to move forward.

Author Bronnie Ware, an Australian nurse, shared her experience working in palliative care with patients who only had weeks to live. She found they had a clearer perspective about life.

When asked if they had any regrets, common themes began to surface. Among their top regrets were: They wished they had not made work a priority. They regretted not spending more time with friends and family, especially when their children were young. They admitted not expressing their true feelings. Settling for a mediocre existence, they never allowed themselves to become who they were capable of becoming, resulting in bitterness, resentment, and illness. Many did not realize until the end that they could have chosen happiness. Instead they remained in old habits, comforts, and familiarities—afraid of change, pretending they were content when all the while they longed for childlike silliness and laughter. The most common regret of all was wishing they had found the courage to live life true to themselves instead of the life others expected. Bronnie reflects, "When people realize that their life is almost over and look back with clarity on it, it is easy to see how many dreams have gone unfulfilled. Most people had not honored even half of their dreams and had to die knowing that it was due to choices they had made, or not made. Health brings a freedom very few realize, until they no longer have it."

Remembering where you began the journey and reading through the reasons to change your life (often) will keep you motivated throughout your weight loss phase and also assist you as you journey on into long-term maintenance. When we begin to forget our distress in the land of slavery, we may be tempted to return once again to the land of Egypt. Let's move forward without regrets.

What does my life look like right now?

....
....
....
....
....
....
....
....
....
....
....
....
....
....
....
....
....
....
....
....
....
....

What do I want my life to look like?

....
....
....
....
....
....
....
....
....
....
....
....
....
....
....
....
....
....
....
....
....

Out of Obesity by Julia Holloman

CHAPTER 7

The Cost of Living

**To fear is one thing. To let fear grab you by
the tail and swing you around is another.**

Katherine Paterson

Historians don't agree how long the Israelites were in slavery, but
we do know they were in Egypt for 400 years and it was only after they
started to increase in number, that their lives began to be threatened.

Similar to living life in slavery, living in obesity comes with
many life-long hardships. As we grow heavier we also face the
life-threatening consequences of disease. However, leaving means
moving from familiar comforts and facing the unknown—in a new
land, with a new diet, and a new set of challenges.

I'm sure that the Israelites were also dreaming of the day
their freedom would come, but I'm certain that they never imaged
that one day out of the blue, Moses would come riding in from the
desert with the news that with their freedom would entail such a
life-changing event. In order to ensure their release from Egypt,
God would send a host of plagues.

Everything in their world that they associated with life,
comfort, and strength would suddenly produce disease and
ultimately death. In the process of exchanging one way of life
for another, they must examine their priorities. No matter what
decision they made, it would come with a high price, tremendous
risk, and a lot of fear and trembling.

> The weight not only stole my freedom, but it determined what I could do and what I couldn't.

At this point, I had little clue what my escape plan would actually include. Even so, I was well aware that freedom would come at a price. Most things in life do.

The price of something sets its value. Even things that can't be purchased with money have a price. I paid a heavy price for being overweight. I wasn't just overweight; I was *morbidly* obese.

The weight not only stole my freedom, but it determined what I could do and what I couldn't. I was growing weary from life-threatening disorders such as sleep apnea, high blood pressure, high cholesterol, and diabetes. These diseases plagued my life and held debilitating consequences. There was a price to pay for prescriptions, medical care, and the adverse side effects of medications.

There are so many things that obesity robs from us. Many of us suffer from back, joint, and leg pain. It may induce life-threatening diseases such as breast, ovarian, prostrate, uterine, and colon cancer. It comes with hormonal imbalances, acid reflux, skin irritations, and hernias. Then there are thing most people don't consider such as stress incontinence, severe body odor, and depression. Many have gallstones, chronic swelling, coronary insufficiency, and heart disease. Consider that fatigue, shortness of breath, gout, menstrual disorders, sexual dysfunction, and infertility are also common. And the list goes on.

Aside from the physical, obesity stole my identity, distorted my personal value, and dictated my emotions. It was a constant source of humiliation and shame. It ruled every aspect of my life: socially, emotionally, and physically.

We may find that we are not too much different than the Israelite slaves. Slaves have nothing of their own, no freedom, no rights, no power, no possessions, and no personal identity.

When it came time for their freedom, they had a choice to remain in captivity under the rule of Pharaoh or they could choose to be free. For the Israelites it meant choosing to go forward into the unknown, in faith, or choosing to stay where they were. If they chose to stay it would mean they would continue to be at the mercy of those who ruled over them, and in addition they would suffer the devastating consequences of the ensuing plagues. Either way there was a price to pay.

The reality is that life after surgery will be different. Weight loss surgery changed my life and it will change your life—for the rest of your life.

I knew I would be going through changes after surgery that would require a long-term commitment towards making major lifestyle changes, but I discovered that weight loss success is about so much more. The insurance company might pay my surgery bill, but I had to ask myself if I was willing to pay the costs beyond the OR?

There is a price to pay for losing weight and gaining life. We need to be emotionally ready and willing to make permanent lifestyle changes. This road is the only one that leads to long-term success. The question is: What will we allow to master us?

My Biggest Fears

Change brings the fear of uncertainty. One of my biggest fears was thinking I would forever be tortured with wanting to eat food and not being able to eat. Which is really not true, but it sure seems that way when you are preparing for surgery. You are told about all the changes in diet and all the foods you can't eat and will never eat again.

Another fear was the possibility of facing yet another failure. I feared there was something seriously wrong with my body that would prevent the surgery from working. I worried that I would forever be left in a state of declining health, horribly overweight, with no hope at all for change. Add to that the possibility of not being able to eat any of my favorite foods ever again, it would be like living in a nightmare. However, in the end, the fear of remaining overweight and unhealthy forever was much worse than the thought of giving up food.

It was really scary to think about such a life-changing

> There is a price to pay for losing weight and gaining life. We need to be emotionally ready and willing to make permanent lifestyle changes.

measure, one that could actually take the very life I was trying to save. Although, I wasn't really afraid of dying due to surgical complications; living with my body the way it was felt like the real death sentence to me.

What if my current and hopeless situation was indeed a forever truth?

On the Heels of Faith

My husband often reminds me that things are never quite as bad as I imagine them to be. Most of the fears I had before surgery were really unsupported. Although I may think I have some idea what lies ahead, I really cannot even begin to comprehend what the future holds. I have found that God always provides for my needs well in advance of my arrival at the next place in life, and He always supplies enough grace for tomorrow.

One of the things I believe about making decisions is to commit it to prayer. I believe that once I find out what God's will is for my life, there is no longer any question about anything that follows. When I follow His lead, He will equip me for the journey and see me through until the end.

While considering whether or not to have weight loss surgery, I prayed, listened, and waited for guidance in making the right choice. But, even so, I didn't have any guarantee that gastric bypass surgery was the right path. But one thing was certain: I did know that, whatever my choice, I had expressed to God my faith in His ability to bring restoration to my life. So, I stepped out on faith.

It reminds me of a story in the *Gospel of Matthew* (9:18-34). As a child, it was my favorite—and still is. It's the story of Jairus and his daughter. The story tells us that Jairus' daughter had just died. As Jairus stands face-to-face with Jesus, he expresses his faith with an invitation—an invitation to *"come."* His invitation expresses his certainty that if Jesus comes, life will return.

Making the decision to have surgery was difficult, and the outcome was uncertain. I believe God always allows us the freedom to choose. In prayer, we too can extend to God an invitation to come.

The answer lies in placing my faith and trust in Him. I have learned from experience that I must trust in what I *do know*, and what I *do know* is I can trust in God. Then, even in times of uncertainty, and even though I don't know what the future holds; one truth will always stand firm. I can trust that His heart is always towards me and that He loves me far more than I can fathom. I am convinced that although He is intimately aware and deeply concerned with my physical condition, His ultimate goal is the condition of my spiritual heart. His heart is to bring healing, restoration, and provision for every need. Every crossroad He has ever brought me to has always moved me toward a higher place.

As Jarius turns towards home, the story in *Matthew 9:19 (NKJV)* says, *"And Jesus arose, and followed him...."*

As Jarius steps out in faith, Jesus follows him all the way to his miracle. Jesus leads, guides, and prepares the path ahead of us, but He also follows on the heels of faith.

Jesus did arise and *"come."* And with him came resurrection of life to Jairus' daughter—and for me, too!

Decisions, Decisions

As I began to seriously research weight loss surgery, I considered the lap-band, which can be more easily reversed. Reversal made the idea more palatable, but after some thought, I realized I needed to make more than just a temporary commitment. Reversal probably wasn't in my best interest. After reaching that conclusion, I considered the unthinkable: gastric bypass.

At the time of my surgery, Gastric Bypass Roux en-Y and the Lap Band were the only surgeries available to me in my area. I chose to have surgery locally, because I felt that local on-going medical support was important.

I spent hours researching Gastric Bypass Roux en-Y on the Internet. I made contact with a few people I knew who had undergone the surgery and had been successful. I reached out to

Over the years
I had a lot of
practice trying
to lose weight
and dieting,
but none at
maintaining
what I had
accomplished.

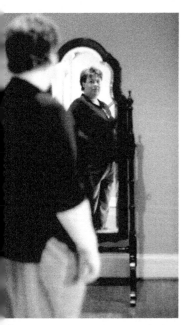

Jan 2006

any referrals they would give me. I wanted to hear first-hand what the decision involved and what obstacles would be in my path. One person offered to have dinner with me, and I asked lots of questions. It gave me a chance to see that it was possible to resume a normal life. The big question still remained uncertain, what was normal?

I needed something that worked. But more than that, I needed something that would last. Losing weight for me wasn't just about *losing* weight—it was about keeping it off. Over the years I had a lot of practice trying to lose weight and dieting, but none at maintaining what I had accomplished.

Weight loss surgery would help me lose the weight and, at this point, it was worth consideration. Deep down, I knew there had to be something more. I just didn't know what that something was.

I did know one thing: if it were possible to lose the weight and keep it off, if weight loss surgery was part of that answer, and if it were possible to find the answers for long-term success, I knew I had enough determination, motivation, and persistence to do it. Somehow I had to make it work. It was my last and only hope for change. I was taking a drastic measure but I was desperate. There wasn't another option. I had to be successful. So, I set off on a new road. I had no idea where I was going, but I did know I couldn't stay where I was.

I set my focus on the unfolding plans at hand, which not only included scheduling an appointment with a surgeon and preparing for surgery, but also planning for two weddings.

It was January 2006. Our two sons were engaged and planning weddings for June and September. Waiting to get started would not get me into a Mother of the Groom dress on time. I didn't just need dresses for the two wedding days, but I needed outfits for all the pre-wedding events. These were the kind of events that you look forward to since the birth of your children. I wasn't about to show up the way I was.

I wasn't having surgery just to be thinner before the weddings. But the thought of getting into smaller dresses did serve as a great inspiration and kept me focused, encouraged, and motivated. It gave me something to look forward to and a chance to look to the future with a new hope that things could be different.

After all, weddings bring the possibility of a growing family. Not only would I have two new daughters to welcome into the family, there just might be the someday promise of a few grandchildren. I had a renewed desire for health and life. Grandbabies require laps on which to snuggle and I didn't have one.

I still had lots of unanswered questions, but time was ticking. I had to make a decision. So, after much consideration, I called and scheduled an appointment to attend an orientation at the office of a reputable bariatric surgeon. I had heard that the pre-surgery qualification process could take up to a year. It might be months before I met with a nutritionist and even longer before a surgery date could be scheduled.

Yet, I didn't have much time. Soon I would need to start shopping for a dress. Thinking about the weddings and all that would come after them, I made up my mind to be a size smaller by the first wedding in June. So with a little bit of wishing and hoping and thinking and praying and a whole lot of determination and motivation, I did the craziest thing. Yes, I did the unthinkable. I went in search for a new diet. It was all I knew and if there was one thing I could do, it was diet. Surgery would help, but it wouldn't come soon enough to get me into that perfect dress. With the possibility of an upcoming solution, I was determined not to lose another moment. I had things to do and places to go, and I had it in me to give it one more try. This time it would be for keeps.

I needed something that worked. But more than that, I needed something that would last.

Out of Obesity by Julia Holloman

CHAPTER 8

Taking the Easy Way Out?

**Behold the turtle. He makes progress
only when he sticks his neck out.**

James Bryant Conant

The next step was to understand what the physical aspects of weight loss surgery entailed.

This pre-surgical process included:

- Locating a surgeon
- Being united with a team of professionals who would walk me through the pre-surgical requirements
- Undergoing medical testing
- Understanding the risks involved in surgery
- Understanding the physical requirements and dietary guidelines
- Undergoing psychological evaluations
- Understanding social and emotional changes
- Choosing the surgery that best fit my needs
- Reviewing financial cost, applying for insurance benefits, (or for some: applying for financial assistance)
- Making the necessary lifestyle changes to support my choice

This pre-surgery period allowed me the opportunity to practice some of the new dietary guidelines, build new mindsets, and establish new eating habits, as well as other valuable information that would help me in making the necessary lifestyle changes required post-surgery.

Wait a minute. What was that again? Did I just mention a diet? I know it seems like an oxymoron, upside down, backwards, twisted, completely insane, ludicrously ridiculous, mindlessly absurd, comically preposterous, extraordinarily outlandish, purely outrageous, extremely bizarre, hopelessly impossible, hilariously nonsensical, downright unreasonable, gigantically paradoxical, not to mention...just plain crazy, but most weight loss surgery patients are asked to lose weight pre-surgery.

I know what you're thinking: *"Pardon me, but it seems to me that if, in fact, I could lose weight, I would not be considering surgery in the first place! Right? Diets are hard. No, more like, impossible!"*

It may seem crazy (and impossible) but a diet may just be what the doctor orders. I had a head start by beginning a diet earlier and I found it served a very important purpose. As for doing the impossible, don't worry, your surgeon can offer solutions to get you started. As for the difficult part, well, what can I say; if you think diets are difficult, wait 'till you take a look at weight loss surgery and what it takes to qualify—not to mention what life holds after surgery.

Everyone knows that dieting isn't easy. It comes with its own set of emotional, physical, and social stresses as you swing from over-indulgence to total deprivation.

While your physical body goes through withdrawal—your emotional state follows suit.

Some people are under the impression that weight loss surgery is easier than dieting. Mentioning surgery as "the easy way out" to a weight loss surgery patient, could set one up for an extreme altercation—there is no better way to get a weight loss surgery patient's dander up (and with good reason).

It may seem easy to leave one miserable life behind and wake up in another, but it's not quite that simple. Weight loss surgery is not as simple as clicking your ruby red slippers and waking up in the world of the thin, fit, and healthy. It seems as though your body and mind are hurled into a violent twister, and you wake up in a whole new world, the likes of which you have never seen before. With all the tests, evaluations, rules, do's and don'ts, and after surgery transitions, you'll soon learn: *"You're not in Kansas anymore!"* It takes a lot of work to stick to the yellow brick road that will lead you home to weight loss success.

Let's just take a look at the surgical preparations, the medical risks, and the changes in lifestyle to see if the unacquainted still agree it's "the easy way out".

What follows is an account of my journey; yours could look a little different.

Finding a Surgeon

My first order of business was to find a surgeon, schedule an appointment, and attend an orientation.

Choosing a surgeon was not just about finding someone to perform surgery. The surgical center I chose included a team of professionals that walked me through the entire process from pre-surgical decisions to the post-operative long-term follow-up care. (To avoid confusion, we will discuss the *post-surgical* phase in more detail in a later chapter.)

That's why I didn't want just *any* surgeon, but a board-certified, experienced bariatric surgeon—one who had a reputation for being sympathetic to patient needs and was well versed in a variety of surgical procedures. I chose a Bariatric Surgery Center of Excellence.

What is a Bariatric Surgery Center of Excellence?

The American Society for Metabolic and Bariatric Surgery sets forth recommendations, and guidelines for Bariatric Surgery Centers of Excellence (BSCOE), even so, pre-surgical and post-surgical guidelines vary from surgeon to surgeon and by the type of bariatric procedure you select. It is important to follow the guidelines you are given by your surgeon.

Finding a surgeon and a hospital that has been designated as a Center of Excellence, or more specifically as an American Society for Metabolic and Bariatric Surgery (ASMBS) Bariatric Surgery Center of Excellence (BSCOE) ensures that you will receive high quality medical care. Centers earn this title by providing a high level of excellence. Through the BSCOE program, ASMBS, and the Surgical Review Corporation (SRC) have established the gold standard in bariatric surgery and are producing information that saves lives.

A center of excellence is not based on the size of surgical group of doctors, hospital facility, or advertising dollars. It instead reflects the surgeons, hospitals and staff who are dedicated to the mission and support of the bariatric program. This title isn't a right; it has to be earned.

There are specific criteria that a bariatric program must meet to be designated as a Bariatric Surgery Center of Excellence (BSCOE) by the American Society for Metabolic and Bariatric Surgery (ASMBS) and Surgical Review Corporation (SRC) which is the independent organization that administers the program on behalf of the ASMBS.

Facilities must have a commitment to the highest levels of medical staff and administration, for the care of bariatric patients. Everyone who comes into direct contact with bariatric patients, from nurses to radiologists, must have specialized training and an understanding of how to deliver care with compassion and skill.

Surgeons must have performed at least 125 bariatric cases in their lifetime with at least 50 cases within a 12-month period. Research shows that surgeons who perform more than 125 surgeries in their lifetime have better results and fewer mortalities, reoperations, and revisions than other surgeons.

The program must have a designated physician Medical Director for bariatric surgery. This ensures that the bariatric program is well represented at the highest level of the institution and it demonstrates that the program is a vital component of comprehensive patient care.

The hospital must maintain a full line of staff experienced in the urgent treatment and management of bariatric surgery complications. This includes an advanced cardiac life support (ACLS) and a qualified physician on site at all times. Further, a multidisciplinary team of specialists such as endoscopists, cardiologists, anesthesiologists and pulmonologists must be available within 30 minutes.

The hospital must have a full line of equipment, instruments and other suitable facilities specifically designed for the comfort and safety of morbidly obese patients. Staff must be trained on how to use the equipment without injuring the patient or themselves.

The BSCOE program also requires that surgeons don't just do bariatric surgery, they must also specialize in it. Surgeons must have appropriate board certification. Centers must have coverage when the surgeon is not available and covering surgeons are required to be board certified, keep up with continuing education in bariatric surgery, and assist in a significant number of surgical procedures.

The hospital and surgeons must use standardized orders and clinical pathways for all procedures. This helps ensure everyone who comes into direct contact with the patient understands the expected course of care, which is important because the staff can recognize when something unusual occurs and respond quickly.

Centers must provide ongoing education to those who elect to have bariatric surgery. Success is a joint effort between patients and care providers. Nutritional needs, importance of exercise and behavior modification, such as addictions, recovery, self-esteem, body image, relationships, and spiritual issues are all components of ensuring safe and appropriate weight loss and long-term weight management success.

The bariatric surgery program must have organized and supervised support groups for all patients. The more support patients receive the more lasting success they will have. Support groups must have a licensed health care professional in attendance to address concerns and questions.

The hospital and surgeons must provide long-term patient follow-up. Tracking surgical outcomes ultimately improves bariatric surgery, establishing more rigorous criteria to become a BSCOE as well as helping to identify the most safe bariatric surgery procedures.

I chose bariatric surgeon, Dr. David R. Miles at Miles Surgical, in Wilmington, NC. Miles Surgical is a Bariatric Surgery Center of Excellence and I was extremely confident in the outstanding professional medical care provided by Dr. Miles and the staff at Miles Surgical as well as by New Hanover Regional Medical Center.

Pre-Surgery Preparations and Orientation

And so began the orientation and surgery preparation process. My first visit included a medical evaluation, medical history, dieting history, and a weigh-in. This process also included learning how eating directly affects one's health, understanding surgery details, understanding surgery risks, and understanding the need for permanent lifestyle changes.

Pre-Surgical Testing

As a general rule, establishing eligibility for weight loss surgery is based on several criteria including weight or body mass index (BMI), co-morbidities (combination of weight-related diseases), age, dieting history, and overall health.

I had several medical tests to assess my overall health and to determine if I was healthy enough to undergo a weight loss surgery procedure.

A full blood panel for blood counts, electrolytes, thyroid levels, liver enzymes, lipid profiles, and a possible glucose tolerance test are among about 20 blood chemistry values and tests that could be performed.

Some patients could have health issues that must be investigated to rule out further complications or pending risk.

My screening included visits to cardiac and pulmonary specialists. It included x-rays, abdominal scans, an electrocardiogram, test for blood clots, and a gallbladder ultrasound.

For most patients, a test for sleep apnea is likely. I had been diagnosed with sleep apnea several years earlier and was fully compliant with my Continuous Positive Airway Pressure (CPAP) machine. Being tested for sleep apnea is not just busy work in preparation for weight loss surgery. Sleep apnea can be fatal. It is a serious health risk and results in low metabolism and ineffective weight loss. It affects your long-term weight loss success, your overall health, and the length and quality of life. Sleep apnea can put you at risk for liver disease, heart disease, heart attacks, diabetes, high blood pressure, and other health risks. Its risks are considered to rank with smoking, obesity, high cholesterol, and high blood pressure. There are several types of sleep apnea (two out of three of these types are not *caused* by obesity) and while episodes may be lessened after weight loss, losing weight is **not** considered a cure. Returning to good health requires treatment for sleep apnea (most likely long-term).

Bone Up

Although some pre-surgical tests are standard and mandatory, you might want to consider asking your healthcare professional about getting a "bone mineral density test". One of the most standardized tests for measuring bone density is called a Dual X-ray Absorptiometry (DXA). This test measures density of the hip and spine and is quick and easy. It does require a prescription from your doctor, however. Bone density is usually a comparative, and it helps to have a baseline to know how your bones are doing after any mal-absorption surgery.

Studies show that gastric bypass surgery can increase the risk of bone loss. That is why it is important to get proper nutrition and supplements. Absorption of calcium and vitamins is essential to insure healthy bones. Getting proper nutrition, protein, adequate water, and enough exercise will be important for bone health along with strengthening muscles and will increase the body's ability to retain muscle mass. Professionals report that preventing loss of muscle mass is the number one way to keep our bones strong, keep us healthy, and help our body from experiencing the affects of aging. I've seen first-hand how broken bones can affect the elderly and their way of life. As we grow older, having unhealthy, weak, or broken bones can change our entire life or even shorten it.

Surgery Risks

Surgery itself carries risks. For obese patients, surgery is a little more complicated and carries more risk than for the average person. Weight loss surgery not only carries with it the routine risk of wound infection, but also the additional risk that comes from being not just overweight, but obese or morbidly obese. Patients are most likely to have several co-morbidities or combination of diseases.

The danger of blood clots and deep-vein thrombosis (DVT) is elevated in bariatric surgeries. We become increasingly more at risk as we grow heavier. This is another reason why losing weight before surgery lowers the likelihood and threat. My surgeon also prescribed a medication just prior to surgery to further reduce the risk of blood clots.

Reducing the risk of blood clots also entailed getting off hormones or Hormone Replacement Therapy. It is thought that hormones may elevate your risk of developing DVT. Getting off hormones drove me a little whacky.

Creating new outlets for the stomach to empty into the intestines, on both ends, increases complications. Early risk after bariatric surgery may include an anastomotic leak, a pulmonary embolism, gastrointestinal hemorrhages, and respiratory insufficiency. These complications can be life-threatening. Post-surgery risks include incision hernias, bowel obstruction, internal hernias, strictures, and marginal ulcers.

Strictures

During RNY (Gastric Bypass Surgery), the stomach is made smaller by stapling. Part of the small intestine is bypassed. The small intestine is then reattached to the smaller stomach. There is a small opening called a *stoma* between the stomach and the small intestine. Right after surgery, it is normal to have some swelling at the site of the stoma. As the wounds heal, scar tissue may develop at the site. Normally this is not significant enough to cause any problems, however, the scar tissue can cause the stoma to significantly narrow, making it difficult for food or even liquids to pass through into the small intestine. In some cases, the opening can close completely. This is known as a *stricture*. These are not uncommon. Symptoms are vomiting every time you eat, even if you are eating slowly and chewing well. Although vomiting is not uncommon after weight loss surgery, it may be a sign of a stricture. Strictures are serious complications and symptoms should be reported immediately, in order to be treated by your surgeon.

The risk associated with any kind of surgery for obesity is harder to justify because weight loss surgery is an elective procedure. Although the array of testing may vary from surgeon to surgeon, these test are extremely important for your safety. This is why your surgeon jumps through all those hoops to earn— and maintain—the ASMBS Bariatric Surgery Center of Excellence designation. Would we expect or desire any less? These additional risks for weight loss surgery are why I felt it was important to find a bariatric center of excellence that could help me make an informed decision before surgery and provide information that would further my chances for success and long-term health.

Meet Your Liver

That leads us back to the dreaded "D" word. Almost every weight loss surgery patient is asked to lose weight before surgery. Yes, there is a pre-surgery diet. Losing weight before surgery is necessary for several reasons: lowering your BMI, preparing internal organs for surgery (namely the liver), and preparing for the major lifestyle changes after surgery. Some insurance companies may require a period of weight loss to qualify for benefits. This is where I was ahead of the game by beginning a diet a few weeks earlier.

I will confess, I had never given a lot of thought to my liver. Why in the world should I care about my liver? The liver lies in front of the stomach, where the procedure is to be done. Losing weight before surgery (even 10 to 15 pounds) means losing fat, which starts in the liver. Shrinking the liver means more room for the surgical team to do their job, less complexity during the procedure, less risk of complications, and less time in surgery. During my office visits, I experienced plenty of prodding and poking on the stomach to determine if my liver was small enough to lower my risk of surgical complications while in the OR.

Gallstones

Gallstones form when there is an imbalance in bile, which occurs when people are on very restrictive diets. This can occur prior to surgery or after having weight loss surgery. During pre-surgery testing, your gallbladder will be examined for health and function. If your gallbladder needs to be removed it can be done during the weight loss surgery procedure.

Studies have shown that 30 percent of gastric bypass patients will develop gallstones, 10 percent of patients develop symptoms requiring surgical gall bladder removal, and 11 percent of Lap Band patients require gall bladder removal post-op.

Your surgeon may opt to remove the gallbladder during weight loss surgery. The decision whether or not to remove the gallbladder should be discussed with your surgeon.

After bariatric surgery, a medication to prevent gallstones, may be prescribed. Taking medication helps prevent gallstone formation 98 percent of the time.

Pre-Surgical Dietary Changes

Learning the ropes for pre-surgery weight loss didn't just prepare my liver for surgery, it helped me adjust to what would be my long-term post-surgical way of life. During this pre-operative experience, I met with a nutritional counselor who helped me understand and incorporate necessary pre-surgical changes and prepare for post-surgical changes.

My new pre-surgical dietary guideline was referred to as "lean and green." I started to eliminate refined and simple carbohydrates (goodbye to rice, pastas, sweets, and fried foods) and introduced more lean proteins and green vegetables (hello to roasting, steaming, baking, and sautéing.)

Preparations for taking care of an altered anatomy also means giving up several items, which negatively affect your new altered stomach, called a "pouch". You will want to wean off caffeine, nicotine, carbonated beverages, and alcohol.

Lights Out

It is never easy to quit an addiction. But, if you smoke, stopping is advised. A study presented by the American Society of Anesthesiologists reported that patients who do not quit smoking before surgery are 57 percent more at risk of cardiac arrest, 80 percent more at risk of heart attack, 73 percent more at risk of stroke, and double their risk of developing pneumonia after surgery.

Smoking increases your surgery risk and slows down the healing process. In addition, it creates an acidic environment for the body, which can compromise your new pouch by putting you at risk for developing ulcers. Your new pouch will be very tiny; which makes ulcers a serious concern for RNY patients.

The benefits of quitting smoking are immediate and significant. According to research, smokers who successfully quit prior to surgery had 41 percent fewer healing complications. This percentage goes up by 19 percent each week a person is smoke-free prior to surgery. After quitting, nicotine leaves the body within 8 to 12 hours. Within 12 to 24 hours, there is a decrease in the amount of carbon monoxide present in the body, allowing more oxygen into the bloodstream. The body's ability to heal will greatly increase between 4 to 8 weeks. When smokers quit 10 full weeks before surgery, the post-operative complication rate is virtually identical to the rate of non-smokers.

The Waiting Room

Did I mention the waiting? During this pre-surgery phase, three office visits were scheduled with the surgeon's office. There were visits with the team of nurses, physician's assistants, and insurance consultants. There are appointments with doctors, specialists, technicians, dietitians, and psychologists.

This means: waiting for appointments; waiting for test results; waiting to meet insurance requirements and coverage fulfillments; waiting for insurance approval; and waiting for the miracle of weight loss to suddenly happen.

The list also included waiting to meet the surgeon and waiting to discuss surgery options. I did not meet face-to-face with, or talk to, a surgeon until much later in this pre-op schedule. I had not completely decided whether weight loss surgery was a realistic consideration for me, which surgical procedure best met my need, if insurance would cover the cost, or if it was even affordable to pay out-of-pocket until the end of the pre-surgery process. After meeting with the surgeon, we decided (*together*) which procedure was best suited to my particular medical need.

And then, last but not least, I waited for a surgery date.

It is a time of informational, emotional, and mental overload. It is enough to make you want to drown your emotions in a huge slice of chocolate cake or munch your way through a big bag of chips. But wait. No, that won't work.

Dealing with the Emotional Stress

This emotional roller coaster is not for the weak of heart. Not only is there the stress of dieting, preparing for surgery, and your own concerns about the risk of surgery, now add emotional stresses from all the naysayers and all those well-meaning family members, friends, and passers-by who must now relay to you their uneducated and unsolicited opinion of what you *"must do"* and how crazy you are for even thinking of such a thing. In the middle of all this turmoil you are sure to hear that this route is the "easy way out." (Right!) Then there will be horror stories that they know— people who had it done and failed. Or worse. Exactly! Just what you need—an all-inclusive guilt trip packed with anxiety.

Oh, yes. Let's don't forget to add the stress of that upcoming mental health evaluation.

The risks associated with weight loss surgery sound really ominous and they are to be taken seriously. It's not just busy work, and although it does keep us busy before surgery, it's far from easy. When is the last time you did all that before going on a diet?

Weight loss surgery is a way out of obesity. However, it doesn't come with a guarantee of "easy", nor is it a "one-way street". Weight loss surgery doesn't come with any guarantees of permanency without hard work and diligence. There are many changes that must be made for the long-term.

Although it may sound daunting, I had nothing to fear. My surgical team was there to walk me through each step and to help me succeed.

I'm so glad you invited me to be your guide and a part of your support team. I'm here to cheer you through the entire process. Now, let's go see how I can help you achieve success.

> Weight loss surgery doesn't come with any guarantees of permanency without hard work and diligence. There are many changes that must be made for the long-term.

Out of Obesity by Julia Holloman

CHAPTER 9

Clap Those Crazies Out: The Mental Health Evaluation

Why fit in when you were born to stand out?

Dr. Seuss

It won't be just friends and family who question you; you will also be questioned by a medical professional. Before weight loss surgery, we are required to face, what is for most of us, an extremely intimidating interview or evaluation with a psychiatrist or psychologist.

Why? Do they think we're crazy?

No, certainly not! Even though our sanity may depend on a little craziness sometimes, it doesn't mean there is anything to fear.

It reminds me of a children's song that goes something like this:

I've gotta shake, shake, shake my sillies out...
I've gotta clap, clap, clap my crazies out...
I've gotta jump, jump, jump my jiggles out...
And wiggle my waggles away!

It's quite a happy little tune and well, maybe for a preschooler, jumping and wiggling may defuse some of that silly, crazy, and boundless energy. But for us, adults, it's really not that simple. Although, I have been known to try to wiggle and waggle my way out of my "crazies," otherwise known as human imperfections, reality tells us it takes a little more strategy.

The aim of this routine psychiatric (or mental health) evaluation is designed to provide an assessment of our mental or emotional readiness before surgery.

Our society often judges obese people, labeling them undisciplined, lazy, and maybe a little crazy. But, really, we're no different than the rest of the world. Our crazies just happen to be more obvious than some. By that I mean we just happen to turn to food for comfort and to cover a lifetime of hurts, stresses, heartaches, pain, and low self-worth. It certainly doesn't mean we're crazy or any different than anyone else.

The aim of this routine psychiatric (or mental health) evaluation is designed to provide an assessment of our mental or emotional readiness before surgery. (In other words, do we really know what we are getting into?)

From a professional standpoint, the psychiatric consultation is requested for the purpose of assisting in the diagnosis, treatment, or management of possible mental disorders or behavioral problems.

It includes a one-hour, face-to-face interview. This will include the following: patient competency, past psychiatric history, general medical history, history of substance abuse, social history, occupational history, family history, review of systems, mental status examination, functional assessment, and any information derived from the interview process.

It's really a starting point to help us identify how we can better manage the stress of everyday life: hurts and disappointments; excitements and celebrations; and all those other emotional moments we encounter.

As we prepare for the extreme lifestyle change, it also helps us understand that having a plan to deal with life's stresses is in order. Instead of turning to food, we must know how to face these stresses and be equipped *not* to shift our addictive behavior over to other vices.

Q   Do you have a plan to deal with stress other than turning to food, alcohol, drugs, smoking, shopping, sex, or other addictive behaviors?

Not to worry, in the next few chapters I will walk you through some simple steps that will help you compose a plan to lessen your stress and prepare you for this evaluation. Being armed with a plan will also help you recruit a great support team, promote the confidence you need to walk your way to success, and assist you in maintaining continued success after your weight loss is complete.

Let Go of the Old

Recognition and honesty are the first steps towards a new beginning. Our honesty about where we are and our willingness to make changes will allow us to step through this first gateway to change and lead us forward into success.

We will also need to recognize any areas in our lives that we are currently aware of that need adjustments or improvement. As we turn to thoughts of a new life, it is important to let go of the old one. If you have a present or past history of drug or alcohol use, abuse or dependence, it will be important to know what role this might play in the future (given the expected stress that occurs in the post-operative period). We cannot even begin to imagine how much our lives are about to change. Even if we don't currently have answers or solutions to these issues at this point, our honesty and commitment to change will allow us to begin the healing process and move forward toward new freedoms and a healthier future.

No amount of wiggling and waggling is going to get us back to health. It takes facing the truth, finding proper help, and our committing to be healthy in all areas of life.

Q Are you willing to be honest with yourself?

Q Are you willing to get the help you need?

Q Are you willing to make necessary changes?

Q Are you willing to get to the root of why you eat without seeking other means of self-medication?

Q Are you willing to uproot unwanted behaviors and feelings of low self-worth?

Remember, this visit is for our benefit. These professionals are a part of our support team and are there to help us return to health. They understand underlying issues that turn us toward our addictions. They are there to offer solutions toward healing, to make sure we understand what weight loss surgery entails, and to help assess if we are mentally prepared.

Although a delay in receiving a surgery date could be possible, on occasion— rarely do these interviews result in a decline of surgery.

CHAPTER 10

The Real Reality

**Obsessed by a fairy tale, we spend our lives searching
for a magic door and a lost kingdom of peace.**

Eugene O'Neill

Do we really know what we are getting into? Life in the land of obesity may have its drawbacks, but leaving the familiar comforts of home and entering to a foreign land also brings challenges. We don't just suddenly appear in the Promised Land. For even though the Promised Land is filled with everything our hearts have ever longed for, in order to reach it we must face the unknown. Beyond the borders of the familiar lies a strange and unfamiliar world that is far outside our scope of understanding or our ability to conceive. There are challenges at every turn and we must be prepared to face them.

Although these changes will be different for each of us—life, as you know it, is going to be different.

If you think that weight loss surgery is the easy way out and that the weight is just going to effortlessly fall off without any cooperation on your part, or if you think weight loss surgery will fix you, your weight problems and all of life's other challenges, or that you'll be forever thin with little to no effort, and that after you're an amazing size 2, that you'll be happy and love yourself, your flawless reflection, and everyone around you—think again.

If this is your mindset, then there is a great possibility that you will end up right back where you started. This is where the myth that this is "the easy way out" gets started. But once you have the surgery, it becomes increasingly obvious that there is more to success.

So far we've only covered pre-surgery risk and considerations—wait until we explore what happens *after* surgery. There are major lifestyle changes to consider.

> Weight loss surgery is not a diet we can quit when we get tired of it or don't like it. Weight loss surgery is a life changing decision—and it's not just about food and what we eat.

Although we will cover these changes in more detail in the post-surgery section, surgery will require making permanent dietary changes, implementing new eating habits, and embracing the commitment to identify and break negative dependences. Even though weight loss surgery will result in many positive changes, there is a great possibility we will experience negative consequences. It will include accepting the challenges of dealing with an altered digestive system—we will pay the consequences for making wrong food choices or possibly face the challenges of developing additional food sensitivities or nutritional deficiencies. Weight loss surgery is not a diet we can quit when we get tired of it or don't like it. Weight loss surgery is a life changing decision—and it's not just about food and what we eat.

Life after surgery also includes adjusting to a changing social environment. Your relationship with yourself and those around you will change drastically. As you become more aware of your changing social and relational environment you will discover that weight loss may not be the sole answer to all of your problems. All the relational issues, marital issues, and career stresses you have before surgery are not going to be removed with the rerouting of your gut. They will all be with you when you wake up in the recovery room. The only difference is that to be successful, you can't return to food for self-medication after surgery. We become increasing aware of relational issues that are beginning to surface, not only with those around us but even with ourselves.

We will need to understand the importance of exercise, taking dietary supplements, finding a proper support system, and getting appropriate long-term follow-up medical care. It can be summed up with making healthy lifestyle choices and being prepared to assume personal responsibility for our health.

Losing weight after surgery will happen, but reaching your goal, keeping it off, and maintaining health will require more (especially more so after mal-absorptive surgeries). Are we mentally prepared for dealing with hair loss and sagging skin? Even the positive benefits of regaining your life and health may cost you something.

Most people who find themselves here wonder what went wrong. They may blame the surgery or even themselves. Hidden from reality, it may seem as though you have been lost in a fairy tale with no hope of peace or passage.

The bottom line is that weight loss surgery does **not** offer us a *total* solution to long-term weight loss. Weight loss surgery is a tool, and the tool works if we use it correctly. A tool makes a job doable, but it doesn't do the work for us—the *doing* is up to us. Even after weight loss surgery, the responsibility of success remains on our plate.

Patients who reach their ideal body weight and improve their health do so with hard work, diligent compliance, and life-long commitment.

Our long-term success *cannot* be based on the fact that procedures such as the lap-band can be reversed. These changes require a lifetime commitment to change and to finding total health.

Making changes for a lifetime needs to be our first and foremost consideration. After surgery, our success in this endeavor will be determined by our commitment to make *permanent* lifestyle changes and develop a plan for success. Lifestyle changes affect overall health, not just weight. Co-morbidities such as diabetes, high cholesterol, and high blood pressure can return if healthier habits are not implemented and maintained.

Be careful not to judge success based on other people's successes or failures. We don't know all the circumstances. Just because someone else had complications or weight regain, doesn't mean they didn't have other physical or medical complications, followed instructions, or that they were willing to pay the price they needed to find success.

The medical profession will tell you that *most* complications during or immediately following surgery may be avoided by doing your homework and finding a Bariatric Surgery Center of Excellence which provides comprehensive patient education and long-term follow up care. They also report that most post-surgery at-home complications can be avoided by following the rules.

It is important to ask ourselves beforehand if we are *willing* to be compliant to both suggestions and requirements to assure the best chance at surgery success.

Q   Are we willing to discover what it takes to find solutions to life's challenges?

Q   Are we willing to examine our emotional, relational, and spiritual health?

AM I WILLING TO
examine my life

seek solutions for lasting freedom?

Keeping weight off for a lifetime is more than going on a diet or enrolling in a gym class. It also takes more than weight loss surgery. Even though I was diligently committed to diet and exercise and extremely determined to regain my health and to remain in good health, I found it took more. I had to go beyond the physical, to find the answers to why I was struggling to remain compliant. During this process, I realized there was one important question that was far more important than "What am I eating?" It was asking myself the question, "What is eating me?"

I also had to explore other health related issues that were causing weight gain and additional health challenges that were not solved by weight loss surgery.

My desire is to help you find something beyond changes in diet and exercise habits. I want to help you discover changes that will result in lasting success. Life can be different and so much more than endless diets, emotional bondage to food, addictive behaviors, and feelings of worthlessness and insignificance. You can be free.

I can't tell you it's easy, but I can tell you it's possible to experience lasting weight loss, renewed health, inward peace, and a life filled with purpose. The surgery itself is just the beginning. The surgery will serve you well—if, when, only, and after—you determine it's personal value, make an intentional effort to understand what success entails, have realistic expectations, resolve to find the root cause behind what brought you to this place, and commit with determination to apply the principles of success.

Does it require perfection? Certainly not. But these are important truths to consider before you make your decision. If you have tried all other options, it may be an option worth considering.

The most important questions you can ask yourself are:

AM I READY FOR

lifestyle changes

&

personal commitment?

Q Am I ready and willing to make permanent lifestyle changes?

Q Am I ready and willing to make a personal commitment to health?

If you are ready to change, weight loss surgery can be the answer that offers you a new start. Let me say that one more time. When you have considered your options and are ready to move from being morbidly obese to improved health, and when you want to change more than you want to stay where you are, then, you'll be ready—ready for a new life.

And life it is! Life and health. Life has so many great rewards. Most patients say it is one of the best things they ever did and that their only regret is that they did not consider it sooner.

An expert on obesity and weight loss surgery, Barbara Thompson, states in the book *Conversations on Health and Wellness*, that according to research done by Dr. Phil Schauer in the *Annals of Surgery*, after weight loss surgery there is an 82 percent reversal of health problems for those who suffer from Type II Diabetes. Seventy percent of patients who suffer from high blood pressure are able to stop taking medication. Eighty percent of patients will return to normal cholesterol levels within a few months after undergoing surgery. There are significant improvements, if not cures, for those who suffer from asthma, sleep apnea, acid reflux, stress incontinence, arthritis, back and joint pain.

You must weigh the benefits and risks of weight loss surgery against the health risks you face living with obesity and the related co-morbidities. It will be helpful to make a list of the pros and cons of surgery and weigh them against staying where you are. It involves counting the cost and understanding the commitment of what success after surgery demands. Every individual should make an informed decision about having such a life-changing surgery.

We have asked ourselves some very important questions. Finding answers to these questions will help you know if you are making the right decision and if you are ready for surgery. Having a realistic understanding of what surgery success really looks like will help you avoid unrealistic expectations.

Once you have gathered information about surgery and have answered questions about your readiness to face the challenges as well as the rewards of weight loss surgery, you are ready to answer the next question.

Q   What is the next best step for me?

My advice: do your homework and partner with your surgeon to decide which choice is the best for you.

CHAPTER 11

At the Threshold of Freedom

It ain't what they call you, it's what you answer to.

W.C. Fields

In this place of decision, we find ourselves standing at a threshold—the threshold of freedom. Here in this doorway there are other decisions to be made that will have a great impact on our freedom as we move forward into weight loss success.

It is time to be released from the things that have held us in our past. It is time for our oppressors to begin to loosen their grip on us. It is time to ready our selves for departure.

It is here, in this place of decision that our release really begins. For the Israelites, this decision was based on a choice and this choice would decide their fate—it would mean the difference between life and death. Would they choose to remain slaves or choose to be free?

It may seem strange to think they might not choose to be free from their present lifestyle. Although this way of life was uncomfortable and life-threatening, it was also familiar. They had to want to leave. They had to want to be free more than they wanted to stay where they were. They needed the willingness to face their fears and the challenges that lay ahead.

Do *we* want to remain unchanged in our present situation or are *we* willing to face the unknown? Is our present way of doing things taking us where we want to go? Change may not be easy, but is it harder than staying where we are? We must choose.

It is here at this threshold between slavery and freedom, that *our* future is decided and for us, also, it is time to remember who we are or who we chose to be.

It's easy to let others define us. For the children of Israel, this choice hinged on their identity of who they thought they were and who they chose to be. They may have been living in the land of Egypt, but that didn't make them Egyptians. They were God's chosen people, heirs of the Promised Land, and they carried the seed of promise within them.

You Have What It Takes

Maybe I don't know your name or where you live, but there are some things I do know about you. I know that if you are considering having weight loss surgery or have had weight loss surgery, you have spent a lot of time dieting. It means you have been diligent, have demonstrated tremendous willpower, and are fully acquainted with discipline.

I believe that you are creative, resourceful, and fully capable to accomplish that which you set your mind to accomplish. I believe that you know what it takes to be disciplined and are intimately familiar with perseverance. After many repeated weight losses, weight regains, or what you may consider to be failures, it tells me that *you* have been striving to overcome against all odds. You are strong and determined. I am certain that you are not a failure. You need to know that about yourself.

I believe that you want to be different more than anything else. I believe you have a dream, one that you haven't given up on. You might have laid it down somewhere along the way, but it's time to go back and pick it up.

I believe that you are willing to do whatever it takes to lose weight and find health. Just because you haven't accomplished it yet, just means you haven't reached the finish line *yet*. There is still hope and there is still a way to make it happen.

I know that you have overcome many obstacles and you can overcome this obstacle, too.

I know what it's like to be entangled in the bondage of life's circumstances. I know how it feels to seem powerless to overcome them. It is easy to feel overwhelmed, discouraged, and defeated.

I discovered a scripture in *Genesis* (46:3, 4) that says God used the time of slavery in Egypt to form Israel into a great nation. However difficult it is to understand, God uses our struggles and difficult situations to strengthen us, as well. He never promises that we will not encounter trouble. But, He gives us the faith and strength to walk through it; the guidance and wisdom to walk around it; and the power and provision to overcome it. Even in our weakness, He is strong. He holds an abundant supply of grace for each new day. His love and compassion will never fail. He reassures us that He relentlessly watches over us, devotedly stands with us, and whole-heartedly acts on our behalf. If we choose to follow, He will lead and guide us out of the land of slavery and will faithfully bring us into the Promised Land victorious.

I can tell you that all is not lost and the journey is not over. I believe in you. I am here to cheer you on to the finish line. Don't give up now; you are closer to the Promised Land than you think. I believe you can be successful. Now, it's time for *you* to believe in yourself.

It's also time to think about who you want to *become*, as a person. When my children were young, I used to tell them they could *become* whatever they wanted to *become*. *Becoming* involves more than our occupation or what we *do*. It is about who we want to *be*, on the inside.

Your weight has most likely held you back from *doing* all you wanted to *do*. But right now you have the opportunity to choose to *become* all you were created to *be*. Who do you want to be?

Diets require discipline and willingness to change, these we have certainly had lots of practice in *doing*. And, yes, we do need discipline and the willingness to change. But as we all know these alone don't produce the kind of change we need. Diets are based on very good intentions, but have you ever noticed that it takes more than good intentions to transform our lives. It takes more than *doing*. Although we need to make lifestyle changes and rid ourselves of unwanted habits, lasting change must come at a deeper level than physical behaviors. True change is not just about what you *do* and success is not measured in what we have *done*, but is expressed in the wealth of our soul and it begins with who we *are*.

What we believe about ourselves starts with how we see ourselves and what we think about our ability to achieve our goals.

- **Q**   Who do you say you are?
- **Q**   Is the image you have of yourself limiting your potential?
- **Q**   Does the image you have of yourself
line up with how God sees you?
- **Q**   What does God say about who you are?
- **Q**   Who do you want to be? (It will be good to make a list.)

What we believe about ourselves starts with how we see ourselves and what we think about our ability to achieve our goals. It's not just about positive thinking; it's so much more.

With the recovery of *our* hopes and dreams, we, too, must find the faith to achieve them. We must find the faith to leave the past behind in search of a new land and a new you. It's time to discover who you *are* and who you want to *be*.

Within you, is the seed of something great, the seed of success, and it is time to plant it. Your faith may seem small but once you plant the seed, the treasures that await are abundantly worthwhile. Even the tiniest seed of hope holds within it incomparable riches, unlimited possibilities, the promise of new life, and new beginnings.

Success is achieved and maintained by people who refuse to quit. They have their eye on a prize, which calls them upward and forward toward a goal. Do you believe you can attain your goal? How will you achieve it?

Most of us allow negative seeds to be planted in our mind until we stop short of our fullest potential. Don't let fear arrest your efforts. Don't let past failure keep you from reaching your potential.

Failure is not being knocked down; failure is giving up. You know the saying; *"If at first you don't succeed—try, try again."* If it doesn't happen the first time, it doesn't mean it's not meant to happen. It took ten plagues for Pharaoh to release the Israelites from bondage. It didn't happen on the first try, or even the ninth. God didn't give up on their release and neither can you give up on yours.

Don't settle for less than your ultimate potential. So what if you had friends and family members who had weight loss surgery and gained the weight back. So what if you have been on a thousand diets and gained back more. So what?

Many of us have not just stopped with the average weight loss, but continued until we reached a realistically healthy and manageably achievable weight. How did we do it? We believed it could be done, and we believed we could do it, too. We fixed our eye on the goal and determined inside we would be successful. And no matter who else believed it, we believed it.

Isn't it time for you to experience weight loss success? The only thing between you and your goal is the faith you hold within. Triumph starts with believing in you. Grasp hold of a vision and make it your own.

Out of Obesity by Julia Holloman

CHAPTER 12

Change Your Mind, Change Your Life

Whether you think you can or think you can't—you are right.
Henry Ford

I hope you have discovered that you, indeed, have what it takes to get there. It seems as though we are *ready* to move forward. We are well on our way all right. But just because we are excited and ready for the journey, doesn't mean we are fully *prepared*.

It is here that we have to stop and consider other very important changes that will allow us to cross over to the other side.

During my pre-op orientation I heard Helen, the surgical RN at Dr. Miles' office say that we needed to bring our mind on board. At the time, I really didn't understand fully what she meant, but I found this to be true in more ways than one. Changing our thoughts and adopting new mindsets are extremely important. It is like having surgery—in our mind. Although we can depend on a qualified surgeon to alter our body, we are the only person who can change our mind. In order to best position ourselves for long-term weight loss success, it is essential to alter our thinking just as radically as we are about to alter our anatomy.

What does that look like, and how do we do it? I know—you thought this was about the food we eat and having a smaller stomach. Well, yes, that is the first part. Having a smaller stomach will help us lose the weight; but remember, we want to keep it off. We want things to turn out differently than in the past, with all our focus on the physical, which doesn't work alone. So, we need to find what does.

During my weight loss journey, I found it necessary to examine my perspective of the challenges I faced in life. These and other changes in mindset were even more dramatic than my weight loss accomplishments and have been crucial to maintaining my weight loss over the long-term.

Storms of Purpose, Promise, and Freedom

If you are considering weight loss surgery, I'm guessing you are probably feeling as if life is at a crisis point. I have been at this place of crisis. It is marked by a time of intense, difficult, and dramatic emotional or circumstantial upheaval. It is a turning point in time when an important decision must be made which will affect your future.

However, our crisis moments can give us an opportunity to reconsider our situation and change our direction.

That day in December of 2005, when the scale told me I was over 300 pounds, was unquestionably a moment of crisis. I was, without a doubt, in the danger zone. But it was also a turning point for me. And although I didn't quite see it that way at the time, it was the point when things began to change. At the time, it felt like I was drowning in a river of disaster. But, in retrospect, it was really an opportunity for progress and for moving forward in a new and positive direction.

For those of us considering such drastic measures as weight loss surgery, we have gotten to a critical point in life where extreme measures are in order. It is also a grand opportunity to start over. Sometimes, it takes a crisis to jolt us out of our place of despair and offer us an opportunity to adopt a different mindset. Finding a new and positive mindset invites God to turn our circumstances into an opportunity for advancement. I think He is all about second chances! He most often shows up in the midst of the storm.

Before leaving Egypt, the Israelites faced plenty of storms. They also faced intense cruelty and life-threatening plagues. These things moved them towards an intense desire for freedom. It may have seemed tremendously inescapable, but they were protected in the process. The same plagues that served as an instrument to change the Pharaoh's mind, also positioned the Israelites for their escape to freedom.

Life always has its share of storms. Some are just passing showers, but others produce torrential floods, dangerous lightening, and destructive winds.

There is a verse in the book of *Ecclesiastes* (11:4) that says that even though the clouds are full of water and sometimes fall as a collective flood, pushing its way through our lives, knocking down things in its path, when we focus on the storm itself we neither plant or reap.

I found that focusing on the crisis in my life hindered my progress and kept me from planting new seeds of opportunity or reaping the benefits they had to offer. Instead, of focusing on the negative, I needed to shift my attention to the expectation of positive change. Seem impossible? Things are not always as they seem.

You may be asking, "*What possible benefits could these storms offer?*" Storms can bring more than inconvenient and unpleasant weather conditions. Storms signal coming changes in the environment— they offer hope in a time of crisis.

I live on the coast of North Carolina where we often experience the storms of huge and destructive hurricanes. These storms are not only disruptive but can be life-threatening. As damaging as they are, they also provide a tremendously essential, life-saving function by equalizing and balancing the extreme temperature differences on our planet. They serve to eliminate weak, diseased, and dead trees—giving prospect for new growth. They replenish much needed water in years of drought. Even the lightning of a passing storm releases positive changes to our earth's environment.

Yes, the storms of life do bring change, and change is not always easy. Just as storms are fueled by changes in the environment, so it was with my life. Instead of being caught up in a flood of devastating currents, I had to allow this time of crisis to become an opportunity to experience renewed hope and the positive benefits that resulted.

My storms of crisis brought a much-needed adjustment to my environment—allowing me to level out unhealthy extremes in my life and bring harmony to dangerous imbalances. It offered me the opportunity to find a new perspective, refocus my attention on replacing unwanted behaviors, dislodging old habits, and removing negative mindsets. It presented me with an opportunity to recognize and rid myself of unwarranted fears, pinpoint devastating feeling of insignificance, and uproot life-draining hurts of the past. There were things in my life that were in desperate need of an upheaval. They had robbed me of my sense of value and destroyed my self-image. Some had been growing longer than others and depending on the depth of their roots, some fell away more easily than others. But facing the crisis with a new mindset allowed me to reclaim inward health and pursue personal growth, as well as physical restoration.

The storms in life can also give us an opportunity for positive change. With each drop of thirst-quenching rain can come the promising renewal of life, refreshing puddles for our weary hearts, and greener pastures for our hungry souls. They awaken the abundance of new growth, open fragrant blossoms of anticipation, and call forth fruit heavy laden with the seeds of promise. These seeds hold the immeasurable and astounding bounty of a coming harvest, imparting hope for the future.

Q   During life's passing storms will you allow yourself to reap the benefits they bring?

Q   Will you allow these storms to restore your heart?

Q   Do you need a new beginning?

Q   Are you ready for change to come?

Q   Will you welcome this as an opportunity,
        or forfeit it for a lifetime of defeat?

Q   Are you willing to refocus your attention from what you
        have to *lose* to what you will *gain* from the process?

Q   Do you long for the freedom to
        dance and play in the rain?

Q   Are you willing to adopt a new perspective?

Q   Are you willing to let go of the old and
        put your trust in something new?

It's this perspective that will determine your success or failure. This could be your chance to turn your moment of crisis into an opportunity of a lifetime. It time to grab those brightly colored galoshes and an umbrella, life is about to change!

Out of Obesity by Julia Holloman

CHAPTER 13

All Aboard!

**No matter what accomplishment
you make, somebody helped you.**
Althea Gibson

We have asked ourselves some very important questions. We have discovered some things about ourselves that will be critical such as what we want our destination to include and if we are willing to make the trip. We have spent some time discovering some things about surgery.

We have learned that surgery is not *the easy way out* but rather it is a *tool* that will help us reach our goal. We have also learned that surgery itself will not be enough to take us to our long-term destination. Our deliverance will be a process as we transition from our old way of life into the new. Reaching the Promised Land will require that we have other tools for success.

So what other tools will we need to be successful?

The next few chapters will explore three crucial elements that will contribute to long-term weight loss success—a strong support team, a solid plan, and the mindset to work the plan (so the plan doesn't work you)!

Let's start by getting the people who matter most onboard with your life-changing decision. You will need to communicate your intentions and your need for support. After all, it is the opinions of our loved ones—family and friends—which can have the most impact on our daily lives. Although we may have made certain decisions that brought us to this place, we didn't enter the land of obesity alone. And, we don't leave alone either. There have been many influences. Weight loss surgery doesn't just affect patients; it's a family affair and everyone can be invited to come along. Our journey out will be smoother for us if we involve the entire family. Support teams offer us a place to find assistance, inspiration, hope, and encouragement from those who are willing to lend a helping hand, pick us up when we fall, or devote a listening ear.

We know that change is not easy for us or for those around us. Having a support team in place will help make the journey a little smoother for others as well. Not only have we been influenced by others, we carry greater influence than we realize.

Genesis (46:7) tells us that Jacob went into Egypt with his small family, *"his sons and grandsons and his daughters and granddaughters,"* but they left with multitudes, that included their family, and many other people who made the choice to go with them. The ripples of changes can be far-reaching, affecting those around us as well as the generations to come.

Recruiting Your Support Team

I vividly remember the tension surrounding the decision to do something extreme and out of the ordinary. The discussions alone were life changing.

When my husband and I announced our decision to our extended family, most thought I had lost my mind. My mother even refused to talk to me. I was shocked. It was totally out of character for her. For the first time ever in our 15-year marriage, she called and abruptly requested to speak to my husband. *"What is she thinking?"* she asked him. *"Normal people don't do these things. She needs her head examined!"*

No, this wasn't about bariatric surgery. It was about our decision to home school.

The year was about 1990 and, at the time, it wasn't the normal thing to do. Most people, including our extended family, had no idea what home schooling even looked like. They didn't understand what my personal objectives, motivations, or spiritual convictions were for considering it. And no one asked. They just panicked!

Looking back, we just sprang it on them out of the blue. We didn't stop to consider that they had not been living in our home during those two years of discussions and the trauma we experienced having a child in school who was totally stressed. They weren't there in the middle of it all. They didn't know how much research I had done or how many people I had talked with. They weren't there to observe our first grade child so stressed that he was vomiting every day after school. They didn't see him curl up in a fetal position, crying for two hours at the sight of homework every evening. I don't know who felt more overwhelmed, or who cried the hardest, him or me. They didn't watch the embarrassment and confusion on his face when he began losing his hair by the handfuls. They didn't see his struggle to keep up with the rest of the class or see him missing recess every day because he couldn't copy his homework from the board. They didn't see the regression of progress or the fact that he wouldn't even draw a straight line.

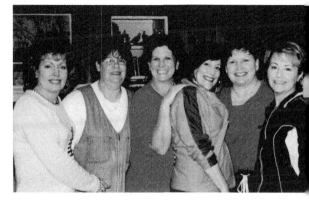

Vicki, Julia, Debbie, Sally, Lana and Vicky

And that was only one child; the other two had their own struggles. The extended family hadn't seen all that had led up to the decision. All they saw was a happy little "normal" family. My oversight left most family members unprepared and uninformed.

This scenario, although about home schooling, is much like what most of us go through when considering bariatric surgery—just with a different chapter title. So how do we handle these challenges? All of us need to feel accepted. We want those close to us to support our decisions, especially the important ones.

How do we approach those who love and care about us with news that is life changing? How do we get them on our team?

Prepare Them

Any good team needs to be on the same playing field and in pursuit of the same goal line. Looking back, Richard and my approach to informing our family about our decision to home school had left a lot unsaid.

Our extended families wanted the best for us. Out of their concern, they expressed fear and uncertainty. They didn't understand the day-to-day struggles, but they did care about us.

Inform Them

No matter what choices we make in life, they always affect others in some form or fashion. We carry much more influence than we realize. What affects us, in some way, affects those around us.

Does your family really know what issues you struggle with? Just because the issues seem obvious to you, don't assume that others understand the full picture. Take the time to inform them about your concerns and the reasons why you are considering bariatric surgery. Prepare them by communicating the entire situation, such as the struggles you are having with your weight and health. Before you hit them with the news that you're considering a life-changing surgery, explain the situation (based on their need to know) and be positive when telling them that you have found a solution.

Make sure you acknowledge, validate, and appreciate their love and concern. Calm and ease their fears. Most of their concerns are likely to be unsubstantiated, speculative, or based on outdated data from the 1980's, coupled with horror stories they have heard about weight loss surgery. Bariatric surgery has progressed by leaps and bounds in education, nutrition, and research since the early years. Be positive and encouraging.

To build a support team, the team needs to know what the game involves: the benefits, risks, and objectives. Information makes all the difference. Inform yourself, and then inform others. Dispel the myths with facts. Express your feelings and objectives.

Educate others on why you are doing what you're doing, not for their approval, but for their enlightenment.

Give them specific ways they can help and support you. Maybe you could ask a friend or neighbor to become a regular walking partner. My family knows cookies, donuts, and candy bars are not allowed in the house. When friends and family come bearing desserts, I ask that they leave with the leftovers.

Do your homework and be confident. Assure them that you are making an informed decision and are seeking professional help. Assure them you are at peace with your choice.

Recruit Them

A good team needs ready players. Team players. Most everyone appreciates being chosen for the team. Commission their support. Tell them how much it would mean for them to be on your support team and that you will let them know how they can support you in this endeavor. They may very well want to support you; they just don't know how.

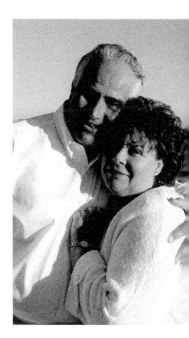

The First Draft Pick

When it came to homeschooling, I had researched the idea for two years before I recruited my first team member. In every major decision, my husband is my first draft pick. If we are not unified as a team, ready to face the challenges together, I know it won't work. His encouragement and support are vital to my success. With all other relationships, however, I took another stance. Their support was important and desired, but not crucial for success.

It was only after years of home schooling that I enjoyed my family's verbal support. It would have been so much easier if they had been on board from the beginning. I needed their expertise and support far more than they knew. I needed their validation and confidence in me as much as they needed to know I wasn't ruining our children for life. My husband and I made the decision to teach our children at home based on what was best for our immediate family.

Make the decision that is right for you (and your spouse) and stand firm. When you say one thing and act another, people see through it. Stand for what you believe. Act on what you believe and know to be true.

All turned out well in our homeschooling efforts. And that little boy who wouldn't even draw a straight line has grown up to be an amazing graphic artist, a talented musician, and a professional photographer. He had a high grade-point average at Savannah College of Art and Design (SCAD), a well-known and prestigious college. He graduated with honors, and currently has a successful career in graphic design. He is a happy, well-adjusted adult, who is a loving husband and father. He is completely and uniquely normal. It's nice to know we didn't ruin him for life.

Most all of my family's concerns were completely unfounded and based on assumptions and misinformation. Our children were not socially deprived. They have success both in business and in their personal lives. We home schooled our three children for 11 wonderfully successful years. We stood firm on my convictions. We enjoyed peace and had no regrets.

Close for the Huddle

When it came to preparing for bariatric surgery, first I sought out those whom I knew would be in full support of my decision. These were my first string, my most positive supporters, my cheering squad, my group of enthusiastic and encouraging cheerleaders, and those who would stand behind me to the finish line. Having this support system in place first helped me to have the confidence I needed. Even though it's been more than eight years, I can still hear my friend La Cretia's cheerful and enthusiastic encouragement when I announced to her my plan to have surgery. *"Good for you!"* she said. It was all I needed to confirm that I had made the right decision.

Then, I proceeded to inform those who were less likely to be positive. I expressed the need and answered their questions. They were very well informed of my decision based on facts and for the improvement of health and life. My support team was excited and cheered me on to success.

My approach was informative and compassionate. I can say that my family really has been extremely supportive. However, I will admit there were some whom I did not tell until after my recovery was complete, and others who were informed only after seeing me 164 pounds lighter.

Group Support

Your close family and friends will be an essential part of your support team, but there are other support members on your team. These include your professional team of surgeons, nutritionists, counselors, as well as local and online support groups.

Studies show that those who attend support groups are much more likely to succeed at long-term weight loss. Support groups are a great place to learn pre-surgery and post-surgery information, but it also offers a safe atmosphere for sharing your personal experiences and concerns. These are the people who know first hand what you are going through and are willing to lend a hand in your recovery.

Seeking out and connecting with other weight loss surgery patients helps us to know that we are not alone in this endeavor. Success. This the goal, and you can be successful. Having a support team is huge during those first few years and will remain invaluable.

It's A Family Affair

It is also important to include your support team in appointments and classes throughout every phase of the process. The information provided during orientations and nutritional classes is just as important to our *in-home* supporters as it is for us as weight loss surgery patients. Be sure to include anyone in the household who is involved with meal planning, shopping, and food preparation.

The wife of one gastric bypass surgery patient spoke to me about how much she learned while participating in her husband's nutritional classes. It helped her to make the necessary healthy lifestyle changes and assist her husband in remaining compliant by limiting unwise food options and keeping the family kitchen bariatric-friendly.

Making changes isn't easy, but we can make these transitions smoother and more successful by informing and including our *in-home* bariatric support team.

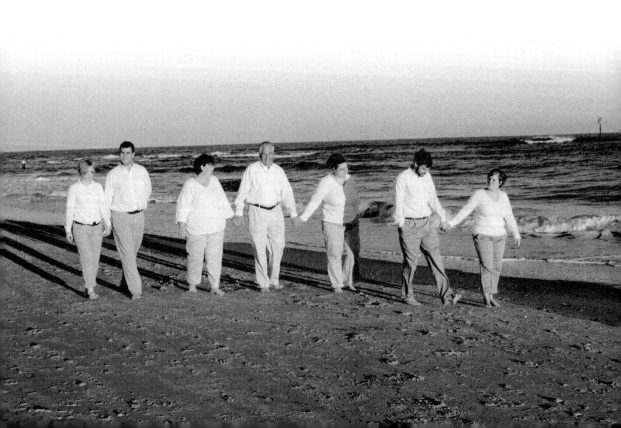

CHAPTER 14

Mapping Out A Plan

I have heard there are troubles of more than one kind.
Some come from ahead and some come from behind.
But I've bought a big bat. I'm all ready you see.
Now my troubles are going to have troubles with me!

Dr. Seuss

The children of Israel went up out of Egypt prepared for the journey and armed for battle. God gave them a detailed, specific, and highly organized plan of escape. This plan included being prepared for the battles they would face along the journey. We, too, must be prepared to face the challenges ahead. If we are not, we may find ourselves facing our former enemies, at risk of being taken prisoner, returning to our previous way of life, or being overcome by unexpected trouble. The time has come to make plans that will secure our freedom.

We will need to be equipped with some tools for success before and after the OR, beyond measuring cups, numbers on a scale, dreams of a smaller figure, and yes, even a smaller stomach or a baseball bat (if it were only that simple). Although, some of these may be very good tools, this task will also need to include a solid plan. A solid plan will help us WHEN (not IF) we face challenges along the way—there WILL BE challenges. We need to plan to have a plan. So, what is *your* plan? Have you given it any thought?

There is a saying that goes something like this: *"When you fail to plan, you plan to fail."* I found that having a plan in place was an extremely important part of my weight loss phase and has further helped me focus on keeping the weight off long-term.

In "Clap Those Crazies Out," we talked about that ominous mental health evaluation. During this visit you will most likely be asked if you have a plan for dealing with life's stresses. Having a really good strategy in place will help make this visit less stressful and more productive.

A solid plan helps us to:

- See where we are
- Keep moving forward
- Record our progress
- See how far we have come
- Stay in touch with our goals
- Know where we need to make changes
- Stay encouraged
- Build our confidence
- Spot obstacles
- Push our way through, over, and around challenges
- Find inspiration and motivation
- Return to the path
- Remain focused
- Overcome
- Keep us from stopping short of our intended objective

PACE

Prepare
HAVE A PLAN

Act
ACT ON THE PLAN

Commit
STICK TO THE PLAN
AT ALL COSTS

Embrace
CHOOSE TO
EMBRACE THE PLAN

A plan helps us **PACE** for success—providing a framework that allows us to create an enjoyable and personalized plan of action that will keep us engaged and motivated until, little by little, we have reached our goal and embraced it for a lifetime.

*P*repare (Have a plan)
*A*ct (Act on the plan)
*C*ommit (Stick to the plan at all costs)
*E*mbrace (Choose to embrace the plan)

Prepare the Plan

Having a plan is like having a map or itinerary. It keeps us on the right path and helps us reach our goals. Every plan will be different, but there are certain basic components our plan must include. It begins with defining our personal goals, discovering our motivators, forming a plan of action, choosing to embrace the plan, and believing we have what it takes to accomplish the task.

Identify the Goals

Forming a plan starts by looking at the overall map. It includes writing out a clear vision of where you are, where you want to be, and how you want to achieve it. Actually, you took the first step when you decided to chart a new course of action. However, reaching goals depends on your ability to complete them.

A *goal* is something that can be achieved by our own efforts. Although you need support, information, and encouragement from others, you should be able to complete the goal without the cooperation of anyone else. Goals should be personal and specific to *you*.

Sometimes we have *desires* that are based on things that we don't have the power to change. We can't control our outcome if we are depending on the uncertain cooperation of others.

We must accept the fact that we can only change what is within our own willingness to change. We can only change ourselves, not others. We must learn to distinguish the difference between what is within our ability to control and what is not. We may not always be able to change our circumstances, but we can make the choice to change how we respond.

When setting goals, we must define the things that are within our power to change and set our goals accordingly. Then our goals will be achievable, realistic, and reachable.

> When setting goals, we must define the things that are within our power to change and set our goals accordingly.

With the list of goals in hand, it is helpful to ask these questions:

Q Are the goals within my power to achieve?

Q Can I, by my own efforts, without the cooperation of anyone else, control the outcome of my goals?

Q Do my goals line up with my personal values and convictions?

Q Are the goals important and meaningful enough to keep me motivated?

Q Are my goals "SMART": **S**pecific, **M**easurable, **A**ttainable, **R**ealistic, and **T**imely?

Q Have I found the support I need to keep me encouraged?

Q What can I do to accomplish my goal?

Q Am I willing to commit it to prayer?

Create Milestones

These life-changing events don't just happen by accident, and wishing things to be different won't get results. It is necessary to make it your focus.

Earlier we answered questions about what benefits the surgery would offer. Focusing on the benefits and rewards this new discipline will bring, will keep you motivated. The benefits must be strong enough to motivate you to see it through 'til the end. If the goal is challenging and exciting, it will push you through plateaus and over obstacles in your path.

The benefits of reaching the goal become mile markers in the journey. These mile markers are short-term stepping-stones that will mark your progress and give you an immediate reward and sense of accomplishment.

I set an overall *long-term goal* for myself while considering weight loss surgery. I wanted to be healthier. I wanted (or desired) to regain my health both physically and emotionally. Then, there were the *benefits* and rewards, such as the possibility of getting off my prescription medication. Although better health was certainly a possibility, getting off prescription medication was not guaranteed. On the other hand, shopping in a normal clothing store, and fitting into a normal-size world were achievable.

The rewards served as great motivators, such as fitting into a smaller "mother-of-the-groom" dress. These were the *short-term goals* that became milestones in the journey. They allowed me the opportunity to celebrate my accomplishments along the way.

I keep several journals. I am a relentless journalist and an incurable list maker. I went a step further than just the notebook; I also got a scrapbook. In the scrapbook, I included photos each month. I recorded my thoughts, feelings, and intentions, reviewed my plans and goals, and updated my progress. It also helped me to review my dreams and celebrate victories—large and small. I collected pictures and ideas that would keep me motivated. I recorded my dreams, such as my desire to work in my yard or clothing I wanted to wear. I reviewed them often. Seeing my forward progress kept me consistent and committed. This also served another purpose—it helped me remember where I came from.

Form the Plan of Action

Now that *you* have *your* eye on the long-range goals, have formed a clear and realistic direction of where you are going, and have fixed your focus on the benefits they offer, it's time to form a plan that will take you through, day by day.

Lifestyle changes happen when we make daily changes and establish daily habits. John Maxwell has written several books on this subject, and he puts it this way: "*You will never change your life until you change something you do daily. The secret of your success is found in your daily routine.*" By focusing on reaching long-term goals and the benefits of the end result, I was motivated to act on the day-to-day process it took to achieve it. Daily short-term sacrifices will produce long-term success.

It's time to brainstorm options and ideas that you can use to make these happen. Your plan will need to be something that works for you. It will also need to be simple, doable, and clear—precise

> Daily short-term sacrifices will produce long-term success.

plans for "hitting the mark." These ideas also need to be exciting and interesting. Incorporate activities that you find motivating.

It is important to note that the plan will require ongoing adjustments as strategies change throughout the process.

You will need:

- A plan for exercise
- A plan for eating
- A plan for when you are tempted to eat
- A plan for recognizing when you are using food for comfort
- A plan for dealing with unwanted eating behaviors
- A plan for dealing with stress
- A plan to keep you motivated and moving forward
- A plan for escaping trouble
- A plan for identifying what is keeping you from fulfilling your plan

You definitely need a plan.

At each obstacle, it is important to stop, evaluate, and make a workable solution that will help you overcome anything that is hindering you from your success. Finding solutions to challenges and obstacles will assure that you are making forward progress.

It's great to have lots of creative ideas in which to accomplish your goals. If plan A fails, have plan B, C, D, and all the way to Z and beyond for that matter. Your list of options can be as long as you need.

After you have decided on the goals and have listed things you plan to do to achieve them, you may find it helpful to discuss them with a support person you trust to determine if you are on the right track. This will keep you encouraged along the way. Having someone to encourage you when you falter and rejoice with you in your victories increases your possibilities and empowers you toward success.

Part of that plan includes having support, and you will get it—from medical professionals, dieticians, your sturdy support team of family and friends, and other weight loss surgery patients like me! But let's not forget the most important support person you've overlooked for far too long—*you!* Discovering who you are and learning how to encourage yourself will be an indispensible asset.

This plan will allow the surgery tool of a new sized pouch to do its part, while you do yours. Working together with your new surgery tool and focusing on the short-term day-to-day steps of your new plan will allow you to fulfill your long-term goals.

Act on the Plan

Having lofty goals and making a great plan is one thing, but you must be willing to put the plan into action. Success at anything requires focusing on the target you plan to hit and remaining on target.

One of my plans was to be more active. It started the first day home from the hospital. I began by walking inside and then progressed outside by making it to the end of my street (which took 5 minutes or less.) Next, I progressed for 10 minutes, then 20, then 30, and then a mile. After a while, I was able to progress to 3 miles, then 6. Before I knew it, I was planning to walk in a half marathon. From time to time I have hired a personal trainer, purchased a few pieces of in-home exercise equipment, as well as videos and recorded TV exercise programs. I added simple everyday things into my routine such as parking further away from my shopping destination and working in the yard.

One of the tools that helps bridge my day-to-day efforts into long-term success is *food journaling*. Studies show that people who keep food journals are more likely to keep weight off long term and usually experience double the weight loss as those who do not. This easy and effective discipline is a matter of habit and provides accuracy as well as awareness that profoundly affects weight loss and maintenance efforts. I tried several methods, from pen and paper to computer programs, but I found that smart phone applications worked best for me.

You can create diversions and strategies that will allow you to both overcome obstacles and manage stress. Remember, the key to working the plan is staying motivated. Once you find a galvanizing focus, find inspiring activities that will keep you engaged in the task. They could look something like this: take a walk, go to a gym, take a bath, read a book, take a vacation, find a hobby, get a massage, relax, and pray. Create an in-home spa, plant a garden, play tennis or golf. Heck, play all day. Take a road trip, listen to music, and while you're at it, take out the papers and the trash, dust and scrub that kitchen floor, just finish cleaning up your room. Let's see that dust fly with that broom, get all that garbage out of sight, you're going out on Friday night. You just put on your coat and hat, and walk yourself to the laundry mat. And when you finish doing that, bring in the dog and put out the cat. Yackety, yack, don't talk back. Don't give me no dirty looks. I'm really hip. I know what cooks. Just tell all of your excuses to take a cruise, 'cause you've got life to live and weight to lose! You'll be rocking and rolling down the highway of success in no time.

Yeah, I'm crazy!

Your list needs to be long. Really long! You'll be adding plenty more in the years to come 'cause you'll be nice and skinny, sporting that yellow polka dot bikini. (Even a pair of shorts would be nice!)

My friend Hannah shared that she discovered some things about herself during her weight loss journey. She found that watching certain television shows caused her to want to eat. She also discovered that the reason behind wanting to eat was that she felt stressed. So, she came up with a few strategies. First, she identified the reason behind her desire to eat. Next, she eliminated the problem by removing herself from the unwanted stress—she turned the channel. She further devised a plan to help her break the habit of eating while watching TV—she traded in the bag of chips for several bottles of fingernail polish. She found that having wet nails and eating chips didn't go together.

> # Am I willing to do what it takes to see the goal fulfilled and maintained?

She did go through quite a supply of nail polish, but it was well worth the effort. Hannah had to find a creative solution to her challenges. You can, too.

Commitment and Consistency

How do you make it happen? By being intentional.

The third and fourth keys are commitment and consistency. This will mean making *intentional lifestyle* changes which require determination and continued motivation for the long haul. Make them a priority and adopt them for life. Even after you hit the target, you can't retreat.

Act on the plan, and don't give up. Although reaching the intended objective depends on making realistic and attainable goals, it also includes a willingness to do what it takes to see them through. It is extremely important to focus your eye on the goal, to motivate yourself, and to keep going. Discover what it will take to help you focus on your objectives, motivate you to achieve your goals, and realize *continued* success.

Earlier we talked about considering the cost involved in making lifestyle changes. AT ALL COSTS, you must be willing TO STICK TO THE PLAN.

I knew there were certain sacrifices I must make in order to get there. I had to ask myself some hard questions. I was the only one who could answer these questions; no one else could do it for me. It was my personal decision based on a desire to change and succeed, my own personal values, and my willingness to commit to the discipline it would require.

> What things can I do to keep motivated?

Q Am I willing to do what it takes to see the goal fulfilled and maintained?

Q What am I willing to do in order to see it through until the end?

Q What value do I place on the end result?

Q How strong is the desire to see my goal come to reality?

- **Q** Is my motivation strong enough to stick to the plan at all costs?
- **Q** What things can I do to keep motivated?
- **Q** Do I believe I can attain it?
- **Q** Am I willing to go there?
- **Q** Who will I need on my team to help me during the rough spots?
- **Q** Where can I go for help?

I had to continually ask myself these questions at each phase of the journey. Long-term success requires a long-term commitment.

Embrace the Plan

One of the most important elements of my success came when I realized I had to change my mindset in order to change my anatomy. Mindset changes are the foundation that will give the plan its stability. I compare them to an umbrella.

An umbrella offers us protection as we move through stormy weather. At first, like an umbrella, your plan will be delicate, fragile, and easily turned inside out by a strong gust of wind. Embracing the plan is like holding on to that umbrella for dear life even when the winds are fighting against you. It's more than just acting on the plan. Embracing the plan requires intentionally adopting a positive attitude, accepting it with eagerness, and purposefully choosing to make it work.

Long-term success requires a long-term commitment.

I discovered that going through the motions would not keep me motivated for the long-term. I had to make it a point to intentionally review and rethink the plan to keep it fresh and enjoyable. A positive perspective promotes energy and includes planning activities that are interesting, exciting, and keep you moving toward the goal. Embracing the plan and being willing to commit to lifestyle changes offers us protection from discontentment, complacency, and indifference.

The Israelites had to make the same choice. They could bend under the fear of the Pharaoh's rule, or they could choose to wholeheartedly embrace the plan that God had provided as way of escape. Although, I'm sure they weren't packing any galoshes or umbrellas in their travel bags, they did need protection through some stormy circumstances, both before and after their departure from Egypt. God promised them protection but they had to continually make choices to embrace the new and leave behind the old.

Although it may be tempting to take a short cut and avoid making plans or changes in mindset, I wouldn't advise it. It may seem like a lot of work, but it provides a very important purpose— allowing you a safer and more reliable journey onward.

God provided an exquisitely detailed plan that allowed the Israelites to escape Egypt. After their escape, they didn't take the shortest route, but rather the long way around. God knew something they didn't know. The Egyptian military was posted along the shorter route. Likewise, the decision to take *short cuts* may result in *short-term* success.

Changing my mindset held one of the greatest keys to my success. As my journey unfolds, I will share with you what these mindset changes involved, but for now it will be important to realize that what we choose to embrace will have a major impact on our progression to success. Like our umbrella, in order to be completely successful, once we have it up and in place, it is our responsibility not to let go. Change will only come if we are honest with ourselves, determined to change, persistent until it comes, and committed to the long-term.

Your plan will take you from small, everyday changes to bigger and more far-reaching ones and help you unlock your dreams of long-term weight loss. Based on your own *personal* goals and your *personal* value on success, having a plan will give you avenues of motivation, encouragement, and the inspiration you need. You don't have to wait. You can start now.

> One of the most important elements of my success came when I realized I had to change my mindset in order to change my anatomy.

CHAPTER 15

The Last Supper

**You can clutch the past so tightly to your chest
that it leaves your arms too full to embrace the present.**

Jan Glidwell

By now you may have heard of the *"honeymoon stage."* This is a
period of time right after gastric bypass surgery when the weight
seems to fall off effortlessly and we're so thrilled we had surgery.
Just like those who are newly wed, life is wonderful. How did we
ever live without it?

Well, there is another stage you may not hear so much about,
but I'll bet my bottom dollar that you are well acquainted with it.

As the pre-surgery phase draws to a close, and our dietary
habits hover on the precipice of the terrifying abyss of permanent
change, panic sets in, and all we can think about are the foods we
will never eat again—or so we think! Our goal in life now becomes
a persistent and unrelenting search to track down and devour each
and every food item that we love to eat. We simply must savor that
taste at least one more time. So we set out on a food binge.

It could very well be more than one meal. It could be every
food item we have ever enjoyed, all motivated by the fear that we
will never be able to eat it again. We feel our life ticking away as we
slowly slip into a deeper depression with every passing meal. It's a
farewell party to food and the end to life, as we know it.

Sound familiar? We have all been here. I can almost guarantee that every diet we have ever attempted was preceded by this outrageous attempt to hold on to that which we perceive will be lost forever—the taste, comfort, and enjoyment of food. It is what many call the *"Last Supper Stage"* just prior to surgery.

Believe me, I understand. Before surgery, the very thought of giving up rice was almost a deal-breaker. I just didn't know if I could go on living without it.

Our eating habits will be different after surgery. Absolutely, positively, undoubtedly, unmistakably, indisputably, undeniably, definitely, and unequivocally, YES! We have to drastically change our lifestyle. But it is not as terrible as it seems. My pre-surgery fears about what I *thought* eating would be like after surgery were unfounded. So, how do we prevent the detrimental "Last Supper" panic attack and gain a more realistic perspective?

> First, it is important to understand that our departure from food is going to be an emotional experience as well as a physical one.

First, it is important to understand that our departure from food is going to be an emotional experience as well as a physical one. This is possibly the single most important piece of information you can know prior to surgery. We can expect to face emotional challenges as physical lifestyle changes begin to unfold.

This last supper mentality is simply a response to our fear and uncertainty as we face unpredictable change and anticipate the loss of food. It is a normal and very real part of the weight loss surgery process. These feelings begin early, even here in this pre-op stage and continue throughout the stages of post-op recovery.

Recognizing these feelings will give you an opportunity to connect with the reality of your changing world. It will be helpful to use this time to accept the reality of living life with an altered anatomy and ready your mind for the changes to come.

Your food choices must change after surgery, no question about it. Depending on how your body reacts to surgery and which procedure you have done, foods such as rice, pasta, and bread may be off limits or very limited for you short term or maybe even long-term. But the truth is, we don't have to give up every food item and taste we have ever enjoyed—forever. There are still plenty of really good foods with great taste to enjoy while remaining within healthy limits. Since surgery, I probably enjoy food more than ever. I've heard other patients say that too.

There will be foods that you can learn how to eat within the limits of a proper carbohydrate and protein balance. When your pouch is mature, you can enjoy many of your favorite foods again, without discomfort, and without gaining weight.

When I was told I couldn't eat rice after surgery, I really thought that meant forever. But that was simply not true. Yes, rice swells beyond the capacity of the newly sized pouch. And yes, for a while I had to nix it from the menu. But along the way I was able to add it back to my diet, in smaller portions. That was when I was experienced enough to know how much to eat and not to get in trouble. I eat it on occasion. It still tastes really good. I don't experience that "I can't live without it" panic anymore. And believe it or not, I don't over-indulge. Was giving up rice hard? Yes, in the beginning. But, it wasn't nearly as hard as I had imagined it was going to be—and neither was it permanent.

There will be food items that will be to your advantage to give up long-term. This will include highly processed and refined foods, and foods that are high in fat and sugar. Carbonated drinks are among the top of the list. I know, you're saying, *"But, Julia, you don't understand!"* Oh, but I do. I used to drink two 2-liter bottles a day of "The Real Thing." Yep, two 2-liters! But I made up my mind to give up cola years ago when I realized that caffeine was triggering migraine headaches. I didn't want to give it up, but my desire to avoid a migraine headache far surpassed my desire for soda. I haven't had carbonated beverages in over 25 years. Do I miss them? In the beginning I did, but not for long. When my migraine occurrences improved, I never returned to drinking them. (I took a sip once, by accident. It tasted like industrial cleaner.) Whatever you feed grows. The longer you go without it, the less your body will crave it.

If you find there are foods that are triggers that send you out-of-control, it could be a while before you can eat them again—some longer than others. Finding new and healthier versions of old favorites or being willing to eat smaller portions is recommended. Some patients experience changes in their taste for certain foods after surgery.

In other words, certain foods will be restricted after surgery that can be added back later, and others you must relinquish for the long-term. Either way, your willingness to accept these changes is crucial. Acceptance will come easier when we focus on the reasons we made the choice to undergo surgery in the first place.

Okay, so you want a last supper. I say, *"Have one!"* I actually think it is important to do so. Feel free to enjoy a meal, or taste several foods you will miss. Do it with a guilt-free attitude. But my advice is to forgo the on-going full-blown buffet binge. Weeks or months of over-indulgence are counter-productive.

In case you're wondering, yes, I did have a *"Last Supper."* I made up my mind I would allow myself one splurge at my all-time favorite family restaurant, Longhorn Steakhouse. I don't really remember the entrée items I ate for my last meal, but if I had to guess, it was most likely a steak and baked potato. The main course was irrelevant. It's the dessert that I will never forget.

I know; you want to know all of the luscious details. This dessert certainly lassoed my heart with a combination that played on my greatest weaknesses—cake and chocolate. It was developed in response to a challenge to see just how many different types of chocolate could be corralled into a single dessert. I think it answers that question quite nicely. Chefs rounded up 6 different kinds of chocolate into this surprising light and fluffy chocolate rodeo which is neither short on chocolate nor on calories. (Don't try this at home folks, it has enough fat grams to take down a whole heard of wild beasts).

Impressively named "Chocolate Stampede," this signature dessert certainly stampedes your taste buds with a layer of chocolate cake made with dark cocoa, a creamy fudge filling with two different kinds of chocolate mousse, and a layer of dark chocolate ganache. It's crowned with an ample supply of shaved chocolate, and if that's not enough to buck you off any diet, it is

> Acceptance will come easier when we focus on the reasons we made the choice to undergo surgery in the first place.

served chilled, with a ten-gallon-hat full of vanilla ice cream, real whipped cream, and drizzled with chocolate sauce to boot.

I got it, I ate it, and I was done. No take home box. My life did not end. This was NOT death row. I was NOT giving up food for life nor did I give up flavor and enjoyment. Was it my last taste of chocolate? No. And, it certainly wasn't my last meal at Longhorn. I eat there often. It was however, my very last *"Last Supper."*

Passover

Having a last meal is not a new idea. The Israelites had a last meal before leaving Egypt. Their last meal was referred to as Passover. This event marked the end of their lives as slaves and the beginning of their release from captivity. It was so significant that God instructed the Israelites to reenact and celebrate it annually. Passover represents a lasting symbol of redemption for the single most important event in the history of the Jewish people. Today, this event is a time of great celebration from captivity, both historically and spiritually for Jews and Christians alike.

Our Last Supper can also mark a turning point in our journey as we move toward a healthier life. Physically, we will never again be able to eat the way we did before surgery. If you took me to a steakhouse today and told me I had to eat a 12-ounce steak, a loaded baked potato, a salad, and a 2,180-calorie Chocolate Stampede, I would be physically incapable of doing so. My new anatomy simply doesn't permit that kind of indulgence. But beyond my physical limitations, the truth is I wouldn't want to eat that meal. For me, my Last Supper marks a time in my life when I was in captivity to my appetite and my emotional hunger. It also marked the advent of a decision to choose a healthier life instead of slavery to the imbalance of over-indulgence and deprivation. I use my Last Supper as a snapshot moment, one that reminds me to continue my walk toward freedom.

Our Last Supper can also mark a turning point in our journey as we move toward a healthier life.

Bypass It

Let me be real clear here, one Last Supper is okay. Holding on to a Last Supper mentality is not. Gastric bypass surgery will require tremendous physical and emotional change. It will be so much easier if you begin by bypassing the old dieting mindsets and begin replacing them with new balanced thought processes. It will be helpful to begin by bypassing the last supper binge and wild swings between over-indulgence and starvation.

The key to a Last Supper is the word "last." Not only is it the last time you will eat this way, it should be the last time you *think* this way. It's better to start on the process before surgery than to wake up to that reality after surgery. Prepare your mind before surgery and accept that life will bring changes. This is a good opportunity to practice getting your mind "in the game," not letting it run wild and crazy. Weight loss surgery allows you a grace period of time when you are not hungry, but sooner or later, your appetite will return. Yes, weight loss surgery requires huge physical changes but it was the mental changes including letting go of the old, a willingness to accept the change, and making up my mind to be successful that made the greatest difference toward my success.

Use this pre-surgery period as the starting point on your journey toward freedom. Your life doesn't have to be about diets and deprivation, or an inevitable return to over-indulgence. Weight loss surgery doesn't mean giving up all your favorite foods forever, nor eating everything in sight before surgery. Eating after surgery doesn't have to be flavorless, boring, or shameful.

Weight loss success is about learning balance, portion control, and healthy food choices which will return us to health. But what most patients don't understand is the importance of changing their mindset. Understanding the truth and facing facts will help you confront the changes weight loss surgery brings.

You may even get to have one or two bites of those sweet treats from time to time. After my weight loss phase, I have been able to enjoy a bite or two of Chocolate Stampede, on occasion. But now, eating chocolate is a matter of choice, as are most desserts for that matter. It is not an uncontrollable urge that rules me. My mindset is that I would rather have better health and be a smaller size than to over-indulge. You can choose what works for you. Does it take time to regain control? Absolutely. It didn't happen overnight or with the rerouting of my interior. It was a process.

When making their escape from Egypt, God gave the Israelites specific instructions to follow allowing them to be "passed over" when Egypt was stricken with plagues. Likewise, I realized I couldn't solve my surmounting weight and health problems by my efforts alone, but I did have a role to play in my own escape. I had to make up my mind to be successful. I was tired of the way I was and I was ready for change to come. I wasn't just tired of being overweight. I was tired of the way I felt when I over-indulged. I was uncomfortable physically and emotionally. I was ready to be free.

A few months before surgery, I began eating very small portions and decided to get serious. Meeting with the nutritional counselor helped me further prepare for the changes in my diet. I focused on adopting an "*I can and I will*" attitude. I resolved to lose as much weight as possible before surgery. I began to focus on what I wanted life to be like and how I would motivate myself to stay on track. Wanting to get into a smaller mother-of-the-groom dress served as a huge motivator.

I made my list of reasons I wanted my life to be different. I developed an escape plan, and began a food journal. It will be really helpful during this pre-op phase to record your eating behaviors in a journal. Become aware of when you eat, how you feel both physically and emotionally, and what you are doing and what is happening in your environment before you find yourself looking for food, and record how you feel after you eat.

I will share with you how I learned to identify and change unwanted eating patterns and behaviors. It was when I became willing to confront these behaviors that I found the answers that allowed me to unlock the core reasons for my food addiction and be free of it once and for all.

The key to restoration begins with release—letting go of the old and embracing the new. Why not let this time be *your* opportunity to celebrate, as you let go of the past? Why not "pass over" the last supper binge and take your first steps toward your new life, now? You can!

CHAPTER 16

Buckle Up

Life is a ticket to the greatest show on earth.

Martin H. Fischer

You are in for the ride of your life. To some, that prospect is thrilling. To others, it makes their stomach churn. It's enough to make one consider other options. It's all about perspective, expectation, risk, and objectives.

At one point, during my fourth year after surgery, I stood in line to ride a roller coaster.

Now, I must explain. For the most part, this adventure was something that was not only outside my comfort zone, it was not even on my "want to do" list. I don't usually opt for this kind of excitement.

Nevertheless, I followed the crowd and joined in. I had little idea what to expect except that it promised to be thrilling, fast, fun, and, with a name like "Everest"—high.

Standing in line, one could read all the signs posted to warn the riders of certain precautions they needed to be aware of before boarding. Most didn't seem to be paying any attention. Maybe the ones who did read them changed their mind and turned back. Some might have taken them seriously because of sound and practical reasons, and rightly so. Some may have been motivated by fear and too apprehensive to even consider the option of going forward. Turn back now. It's your last chance! This ride is not for the faint of heart! But for those who choose to go forward, the thrill awaits.

Two more steps and it was my turn to board. Once I was in the seat and the rail went down, I was committed. Period. No turning back or changing my mind. The track looked pretty straightforward from that viewpoint, and it began quite smoothly. But as I expected, things were quickly going to change. One consolation for me was that I was not alone. As we left the dock, my friend, Anne, offered her support by telling me, *"It's only for 3 minutes."*

Those words helped me through the rough spots. We proceeded forward on our predetermined track, consisting of quick stops, steep climbs, complete darkness, sometimes forward, sometimes back, occasionally slower than expected, then faster than ever. Sometimes I had to refrain from looking down (going up to the heights surely meant a severe drop on the other side, sometimes out of nowhere). At one point, we came to a section where the track appeared to come to an end. But we all knew it wasn't, not really. We had stalled. We just sat there, still. The only thing moving were the "what next?" thoughts that raced through our minds.

Have you ever reflected on your first roller coaster ride, maybe one you took in your early years? You might have begun with a smile, but soon those smiles turned into fright before the ride was over. Near the end, you might have gotten the ride into perspective, as a whole, and probably made one of two decisions: either never to ride again or to go again right away. The decision to get back on was usually based on the fact that you knew what the ride would entail the second time around.

Not unlike the ride of our life after weight loss surgery, previous riders may have tried to warn us upfront of things we might expect to experience. But being so focused on the thrill and excitement the ride promised, we might have discounted the obvious. Some just follow the crowd—it looks fun from the ground. But, beware! Some of those screams are from the thrill and excitement, and some folks are scared out of their minds.

Even though I knew it was high, speedy and dark, the thing about the Everest adventure (like most of life after surgery) is that much of the experience of the ride itself is hidden from the view of the on-lookers below. You see the top of the ride, but the curves, twists, and turns are not visible at all.

Weight loss surgery also comes with some expectations and promises of happiness. But as soon as you're on board, there are unexpected turns and twists. Like the thrill ride of a roller coaster, there is a point of no return. Once you're committed (like it or not), the only thing to do is accept what comes. As with the real coaster, just follow the rules (especially the one about keeping your seat) and you'll be fine.

Having a support team is strongly recommended to keep things in perspective. Just like on a roller coaster, things don't always just go up and down. Sometimes there are stops and plateaus and the waiting gives way to uncertainty and despair. But never fear, the ride's not over yet! It may look like the ride is over and that there is no way through, but going backward is not our best option. That's the crazy thing about coasters: in going forward there are surprises at every turn.

The path may not always be what you expected; it might be better or disappointing in one way or another. Your enjoyment of the ride is always based on what you expect the ride to deliver from the beginning. The truth is, the view is much different once you're at the top than it seems from ground level.

So, before you get on, make sure you have the whole experience in the proper focus. Know what to expect. Talk to others who have gone the distance and have been successful. Have a good support team. If you make the decision to get on board, understand that you must set realistic expectations. They say to those who need to overcome the fear of the bigger coasters, try practicing on the smaller ones. Not a bad idea to practice before you make the jump into the big league.

Once you're on, enjoy. It will be different at every turn. There's no turning back, once you're on, you're committed. Stay the course and focus forward.

When you reach your goal, you will feel exhilaration, delight, and accomplishment. You did it, even if you did scream a little along the way. Screams usually give way to laughter, and after you experience the thrill of accomplishment, don't forget the fun's not over yet. There's always another larger and grander adventure just ahead!

CHAPTER 17

A Personal Resurrection

**And God...Who gives life to the dead and speaks
of the nonexistent things that [He has foretold and
promised] as if they [already] existed.**

Romans 4:17 (AMP)

Remarkably, I lost 38 pounds before my surgery date. People asked me why I would still consider surgery since I was losing weight. Well, yes, I was losing, but the amount was little compared to the amount I had to go. I was still more than 150 pounds overweight. I also knew that I had lost as much as 30 to 50 pounds several times in the previous 30 years or so, and it was only a matter of time before things could change. My hand was on that spring at this point, but with the slightest move it would be out of hand. I knew it would take more to keep me on the straight and narrow. Although I was extremely determined, it was really difficult.

I guess most people would find it hard to believe that, at 300 pounds, I was hungry, but I was. The portion sizes I had to eat to lose weight were not something I could maintain long enough to lose all the weight I needed. I tired of going to bed hungry every night and waking up hungry every morning. I looked forward to the time when I could welcome the new day without feeling so empty.

At this point, the only thing that I was really sure of was that I had tried every option available, and I was ready to try anything to move from where I was to something different.

I chose to have the Gastric Bypass Roux-en-Y (RNY) procedure, which is the gold standard in bariatric surgery, but I didn't choose the date. It was assigned by the surgeon's office. But to me, it was specifically chosen and handpicked by God. It was a day marked by the celebration of new life and resurrection, and it was a day that marked the exit of the Israelites from their bondage out of Egypt. We know it today as Easter.

April 17, 2006, Easter Monday, finally arrived. I held my breath as the final moments approached. I was afraid the surgeon would call with the news that they had overlooked the fact that it was a holiday and would have to postpone. (My first surgery date had already been rescheduled from the week before.)

As I look back, I wouldn't have had it any other way. Even though my Easter Sunday was a only a liquid diet, the fact that the surgery was set for that Easter Monday spoke volumes to me. It was indeed a new beginning. It was my personal resurrection day. I really was being given an opportunity to get my life back. It wasn't until much later that I realized how symbolic my surgery date would become for me.

I was aware that from this moment on, life as I knew it would never be the same. I knew the restoration I had prayed for was just a matter of time.

A Turn Towards Freedom

There is hope and life and a chance for you, too, to experience your own renewal and rebirth. The choice is up to you.

At least one thing is for sure: we have found that the diet road is not the one that will get us there. Taking the new path will be a foundational place on which to begin our journey onward toward weight loss success.

Are you ready for a new life? I am confident that you are prepared for the walk out of obesity and you are ready to set your focus on your Promised Land.

The winds of change have turned our course on the new

path. From this point on, things will never be the same. Say a last farewell to dieting and hopelessness. Set aside past failures and defeat. Tomorrow is a new day and the beginning of the "new you." This time you are going to make it.

It's time to turn your eyes toward your new destiny. The land you seek is just ahead. We are headed home, to the place we belong. This journey is going all the way to wonderful.

We will make our way through the challenging landscape of recovery, and onward to embrace the promises of a new life—a life of peace and freedom from the bondage of obesity. It will be a paradise that expands far above your ability to imagine, wider than your secret hopes, reaching past your greatest desires, and awakening you to a place that will be far beyond your deepest dreams.

The OR doors are bidding us welcome, offering us the long-awaited passage to the land of freedom. As we make our way out of one life, we'll be waking up to a new one—and I'll be seeing you on the other side. Our next stop: life after surgery. Take a deep breath and start counting down from 100...99...98...97....

Out of Obesity by Julia Holloman

PART THREE:

Life After Surgery: Exodus from Obesity

Weight Loss Surgery Phases Two and Three: The Post-Surgical Physical and Psychosocial Adjustment Phases

I am the LORD your God,
who brought you out of Egypt,
out of the land of slavery.

Exodus 20:2

A Chocolate Meltdown

Your imagination is your preview of life's coming attractions.
Albert Einstein

Hot cocoa had been on my mind for days. I had been experimenting with some protein powders that morning and after about four tries, I had finally created one that tasted similar to hot cocoa. Yes, there is an art to adding protein powder into a warm liquid if you want to still be able to drink it. If it's too hot, it will resemble ground-up cardboard.

It tasted so good, like some resemblance of real food. I could only drink a few sips, so I left the unfinished cup in the kitchen. I planned to go back later and finish it. So, off I went to get my morning shower. In the meantime, my helpful husband decided to surprise me by cleaning the kitchen. Not being accustomed to the fact that I couldn't drink very much at one time, he thought I was done and threw away the remainder of my hot cocoa protein breakfast.

Disappointed, I proceeded to lunch. I don't remember now what lunch was, but I do remember it wasn't exactly what I had hoped for. What I really wanted at this point was a fudge pop. Still taking pain medication and not leaving the house on my own, my family promised to deliver some by the end of the day.

Well, by dinnertime, no fudge pops had arrived. They were at KFC getting a take-out for the rest of the family and creamed potatoes for me. I was looking forward to eating the creamed potatoes. However, after a disappointing day and the realization that I was not going to be able to eat fried chicken from KFC, ever again. No hot cocoa, no fudge pops, dinner was late, and I was hungry. It all hit me like a ton of bricks. Life, as I knew it, was over.

Finding myself caught between a multitude of overwhelming emotions and a sea of realism, I immediately proceeded to invite myself to be the sole member of a full-blown pity-party, which took place under the covers in my bedroom with no one around

Out of Obesity by Julia Holloman

to console me. If misery loves company, where was the crowd? I felt alone, overwhelmed, and frightened. I was suddenly faced with the overwhelming reality. *"What in the world have I done?"*

CHAPTER 18

Into the New

**Behold, I will do a new thing. Now it shall
spring forth; shall you not know it? I will even make
a road in the wilderness and rivers in the desert.**

Isaiah 43:19 (NKJV)

Having surgery brings us out of our old way of life. Coming *"out"* of one place means going *"into"* another. Once the weight loss surgery procedure is complete, we move into the "post-surgical," or "post-operative," phase—also known as "post-op."

Post-Surgical Phases Two and Three
Physical and Psychosocial Adjustments

There are three post-op phases. The first two are the Physical Adjustment Phase and the Psychosocial Adjustment Phase. These two are so closely intertwined that it is nearly impossible to discuss one without the other. There are no set timelines for these stages and the pace at which each person will progress will be different.

Transitioning into a new way of life is tremendously exciting. We, like the Israelites, are on the road to a new land. We are full of hope and dreams of living life in a brand new place—a place of health, freedom, and skinny jeans.

But life after surgery offers so much more than this. I can't wait to tell you of the joys that are waiting just ahead. But, as we begin to make physical changes after surgery, there are a few things we may not expect.

During this transition, emotional, relational, and social challenges begin to surface. It won't take long to see how even the smallest physical changes will require new habits, perspectives, or mindsets. The next several chapters will be devoted to exploring some of the things you can expect to encounter on the road to freedom and how to embrace the challenges and the change.

Waking Up to a New Life

My surgery was early that Monday morning. I made it through safe and sound and I was up and walking by bedtime. At first, it was only a few steps to the hospital hallway door. I was a little nauseous from the medication and anesthesia.

I was given a shot of insulin, just after surgery. I took the pain medication I was offered, to stay ahead of the pain, which wasn't much. I also had a pain pump. It felt as though I was pushing the button quite a bit, but the nurse said I had used only a small amount.

By the next day I felt better. There were several tests to ensure I was still "put together" and "leak-proof." Drinking something that tasted like chalk is not a great welcome to a new life and I was thankful it only took a few minutes to drink it. This test was a barium swallow, which is used to search for any leaks in our newly reconstructed anatomy.

Healing became the next priority. I was given a prescription medication to protect my newly-formed pouch during the healing process and also one for pain. A short time later, I was released to go home.

After returning home, I walked a lot. Walking made me feel better because it helped relieve the air in my stomach. I spent my time sleeping, sipping liquid, or walking around the dining room table and the living room furniture. Outside, I walked to the end of our street and back several times a day, about 10 minutes each time.

I made sure I got in my liquids; it felt as though I was drinking all the time. I started out slowly. Some patients find it is hard to get in all the liquid requirements in the beginning, but it is important to keep trying, increasing gradually as time goes on.

Physical adjustments after surgery also include transitioning through several food phases. I stayed on a clear liquid diet for about 2 or 3 days. Next, it was time to progress from "clear liquids" to the "full liquids" phase. Transitioning food phases was really scary at first; but soon my desire to "eat" took over, and I gave it a try.

A Rude Awakening: Here Comes The Pharaoh

As the Israelites travel out of Egypt, God never left them unattended. He gave them a cloud of protection during the day and pillar of fire to guide them through the night. He led them safely around by a desert road towards the Red Sea and they camped on the edge of the desert.

Just like our journey out of obesity, the Israelites experienced many incredible miracles.

The Israelites came out of Egypt armed for battle, but as they woke up to a new way of life, it wasn't long before they faced the unexpected. Pharaoh renounced his promise to let them go and took off after them in hot pursuit.

Not only were the Israelites being pursued by an army of opposition, but stretched out in front of them lay the Red Sea. Having no means by which to cross the vast body of water, it seemed impassable.

I seem to remember them packing a few things for the journey, but I don't remember them bringing along any life jackets or boats, and I don't think galoshes were going to be of any help in this situation either. No matter, it all seemed hopeless. We have all been here at one time or another— caught between a rock and a hard place.

With a huge Egyptian army marching after them, they were hemmed in. Trapped. Caught between Pharaoh's army and the Red Sea. Just when things started to fall apart and couldn't possibly get any worse, they did. I do hope they remembered to pack their umbrellas because there was a dark storm cloud brewing on the horizon and the newly released found themselves in the middle of a raging storm. They were in for a rude awakening. They were frightened, confused, and overwhelmed. I think they were also a little angry.

It was at this point they experienced what I call a "meltdown moment." *"Was it because there were no graves in Egypt that you brought us to the desert to die? What have you done to us by bringing us out of Egypt? Didn't we say to you in Egypt, 'Leave us alone; let us serve the Egyptians?' It would have been better for us to serve the Egyptians than to die in the desert!"(Exodus 14:11,12)*

I found myself in the same dilemma. Even though I came out of surgery safely and fully prepared to move forward, I experienced a few things that didn't quite go according to plan. Before I had time to comprehend that I had just been released to live my life in a new place of freedom, I began to realize that leaving the past behind wasn't as easy as I expected and I experienced a "rude awakening" of my own. That's when my first classic Phase Two hot chocolate meltdown made its appearance.

Meltdown Moments

These meltdown moments are not uncommon among weight loss surgery patients during these early days. They can go on for weeks or even months—and I certainly had my share of them.

At some point, the reality of the situation comes into clear focus. The entire pre-surgery buzz is about losing weight and dreams of new clothes and how wonderful we are going to look in those new size *normal* clothes, as it should, but we are also making huge lifestyle shifts that bring many emotional changes. It's only when the reality of what you have really done sets in that you realize your life will never be the same. We have heard it before, but suddenly experience brings us face-to-face with the hard cold fact—life, as we know it, has changed.

Our diet and our portion sizes have been altered along with our stomach. Our former 4-cup capacity stomach is now a small pouch that is half the size of a medicine cup, which is about 10 to 13 milliliters, or 2 teaspoons. Whether we know it or not, most of us are emotional eaters. Immediately after surgery, it could be four to eight weeks or even longer before we are allowed to eat or chew anything that even resembles our regular solid food diet (depending on your individual need and based upon your surgeon's, or nutritionist's recommendations). Even though I didn't think I was an emotional eater, this was an emotional experience.

After a day of disappointments, the KFC fried chicken was the last straw, but it could have been anything. It wasn't really about the chicken, per se. Not really. It was more about coming to grips with the changing lifestyle. The fried chicken just happened to be the trigger that day. This was real. Food was not going to be the "turn to" comfort and pleasure it once had been. My love affair with food was over, and it hit pretty hard. I had to accept the fact that I had chosen this path and now it was time to walk it. It was time to turn away from the things that sought to take me back into my former captivity and find the faith to press forward into a new life. It was time to experience a parting of the ways.

During this "rude awakening" phase, you, too, may experience a meltdown moment or two, like most of us do early on. As the new reality of life becomes increasingly real, you may ask yourself, *"What in the world have I done?"*

Upon hearing of the arrival of the potatoes that evening, I gathered myself from underneath the bedcovers. With a box of tissue in hand and still in my pajama's, I made my way to the kitchen. Earlier that day, my neighbor, Jan, had called with a soup recipe. I made the soup, measured out a small portion, and stirred in a little spoonful of the creamy potatoes to the correct thinness I needed. If this wasn't good, I was fully prepared for another crying spell. To my delight, it was the best thing I had ever tasted. It helped lift my spirit and saved the day. It might have been just soupy mashed-up potatoes, but to me it was real food again. I really was going to make it.

For those of you just starting out, you can pull through. Go ahead, have yourself an ol' fashioned meltdown. Find a box of tissue and have a really good cry. Get angry. Find a pillow and just have a really good scream. It's important to acknowledge and express these moments as a normal part of the healing process as we begin to realize the impact of the choice we made and grieve over the loss of food.

However, you don't want to camp out here. It's time to accept this new way of life. Once you've had your meltdown moment, and are ready to move on, pick yourself up, give yourself a little pep talk, dust yourself off, and get back on the road to magnificent.

CHAPTER 19

Sea-Colored Miracles

Change always comes bearing gifts.
Price Pritchett

When we last heard from the Israelites, they were questioning their decision to leave Egypt. Hemmed in between Pharaoh's army and the Red Sea, watching an approaching storm, this distressed band of travelers seem to have no way of escape. They were terrified. They thought they were going to die at the hand of the Egyptians. It looked hopeless, but remember that things are not always as they seem.

The approaching windstorm was powerful enough to part the waters of the sea, allowing the Israelites to cross over on dry land. Just as they were safely on the other side, a severe rainstorm turned the dry pathway behind them into a sticky muddy road. As the Pharaoh and his army pursued, the winds began to cease, the walls of water were unleashed, consuming the entire advancing army and drowning them in the sea. God fought their battles, defeated the enemy, and calmed the storm. God had just performed a miracle.

In hindsight, we can all see things from a different perspective. In the moments before, they don't see the miracle, and neither do we. We don't say, "*Oh, how wonderful. A surprise attack from behind, nowhere to run, and a raging storm, thank you God, it's just what I needed.*" They don't consider the sea as an escape route nor do they see the storm as beneficial. They view them as hindrances, and so do we.

Remember, life's storms offer us an opportunity to view our circumstances a little differently. With a new perspective, we can turn our meltdown moments into Red Sea miracles.

These Red Sea moments are places of decision. I faced the same choice. I could focus on the pursuing enemies and the raging storm that sought to compromise my progress or I could turn and face the other option—the sea of reality. Choosing to turn my attention from the things that lay behind and facing forward, allowed me a way of escape and helped me to form a new awareness of what was truly happening in those pressing moments. The pressure of difficult times doesn't feel very good, but it did serve to move me *out* from where I was and *into* a new place.

The newly freed slaves from Egypt discovered something that I discovered on my journey, too. We don't just need to escape the grip of Pharaoh in Egypt, but the effects of tyranny can follow us into the new place as well. We need to be willing to turn away from the things that hold us in the past and try to pull us back into captivity. As we turn and face our new reality, those things will be defeated and we will discover a new path of freedom before us.

These Red Sea moments are places of miraculous encounters. One such moment happened just two weeks after surgery. I was feeling better and was recovering quickly. My husband and I had been invited to attend a dinner party. Even though it was a casual outdoor event, I had mixed feeling about going to a dinner party so early. I was nervous about facing a crowd and food.

I was also excited. It offered a welcome change from the parties of the past, which had left me feeling embarrassed and depressed about my weight. I had lost 12 pounds since surgery, 25 pounds for the month of April, which was about 50 pounds from the beginning of January (including the pre-surgery loss).

I decided to purchase a new jacket to wear to the event, the first new item of clothing since losing weight. Before, shopping for clothes was discouraging, but this time was different.

I was being handed several jackets from which to choose. They were stylish and up-to-date. For the first time in years,

I was actually choosing clothing that I liked rather than just something I could fit into—or rather, something that attempted to hide the bulges.

I recall how I felt when the sales clerk handed me a beautiful aqua colored jacket and I slipped it on in front of the mirror. As I turned around, tears filled my eyes and I felt a sense of something deeply moving. I am not really sure that I can adequately put it into words, but if you have been there, you know.

I was moving a little closer to normal. I was in a store that also carried normal sized clothing, not just an X-size specialty store. Although somewhat smaller, the jacket was still an "X" sized jacket. But, to me, it was like putting on a glass slipper.

That moment was a defining moment. It was more than just returning to "normal." It was overwhelming and it was the beginning of a miracle. It held the promise of something really profound. I saw myself in a different light that day. It had nothing to do with the store, the color of that jacket, or even the size, per se, but more to do instead with the changes that were taking place on the inside and how I felt about myself.

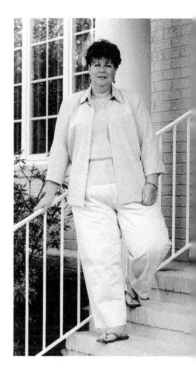

It was the first glimpse of the new me. But it wasn't just the *new* me—it was the *real* me. I had known the real me was hiding deep inside there somewhere all along and she was beginning to make her appearance.

I wasn't just choosing clothing. It was also becoming clearer that I could choose the outcome. I could choose my destiny.

It was the start of a new awareness that this was just the beginning. My life *was* going to be different. That day, that moment, Coldwater Creek became the place of *my* Red Sea miracle. As I turned and faced myself in the mirror, it was another turn of a lifetime.

It was the first glimpse of the new me.

A Time of Rejoicing: Such Sweet Success

For the Israelites, the victory at the Red Sea marked a time when they had to turn their focus from the things of the past and face the things that were ahead. They had to have the faith to cross over to a new way of life. The enemy that pursued them had been defeated and it was a time of unparalleled victory, celebration, and rejoicing as they waved good-bye to their former way of life.

After such a miraculous victory, the past behind them seemed of little concern. With their hopes high, their freedom secure, and their destiny certain, they were confident that the way ahead would easily *"melt away"* before them.

I was experiencing some incomparable successes of my own. In the months that followed there were so many changes taking place. Life was full of excitement and filled with many thrilling milestones. It was a whirlwind of a first year.

I recorded and celebrated the big adjustments as well as little accomplishments of progress in my journal. There were many changes happening and I didn't want to forget a moment of it. Even the small, seemingly insignificant things were very big milestones.

At the beginning of the year 2006, my starting weight was 302 pounds. My pants, a size 26, were very tight.

My surgery date was April 17th.

Before leaving the hospital, I was taken off my medication for pre-diabetes.

The following week, I went to the gym for a 20-minute bike ride.

Soon I began to progress to pureed foods such as applesauce, creamed soups, yogurts, and even Wendy's chili.

I recorded my daily walks.

In May, I added real solid food to my diet. It was my first attempt at making lasagna, bariatric style. I was able to eat half of a lasagna noodle with no problem. Yeah!

In June, the first wedding was all a buzz with wedding showers, and I was 70 pounds lighter. I did get into a smaller mother-of-the-groom dress, and it was a MUCH smaller size. The wedding was in Kansas. My first flight marked another milestone, not having to ask for a seat belt extension.

In July, I recorded that my watch was getting too big and that I was able to wear, for the first time in years, a bangle

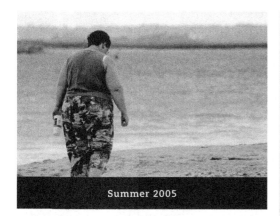

Summer 2005

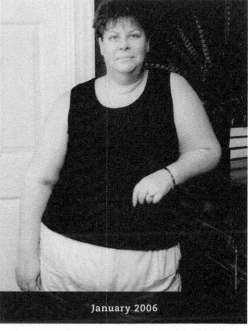

January 2006

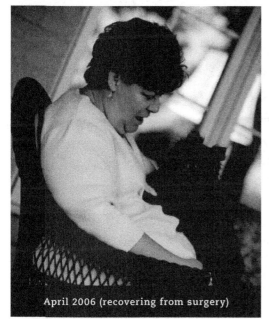

April 2006 (recovering from surgery)

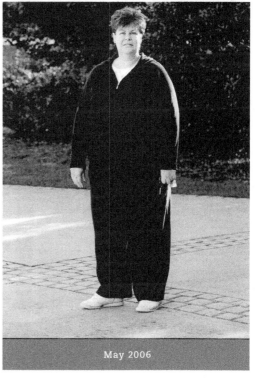

May 2006

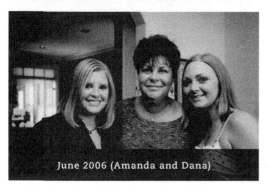

June 2006 (Amanda and Dana)

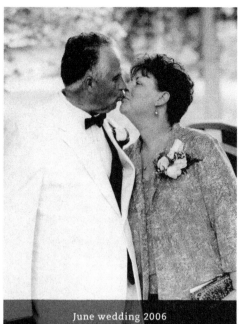
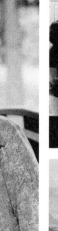

June wedding 2006

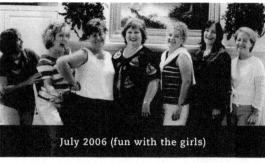

July 2006 (fun with the girls)

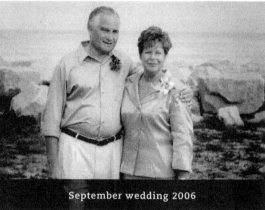

September wedding 2006

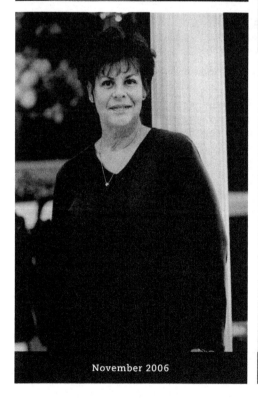

November 2006

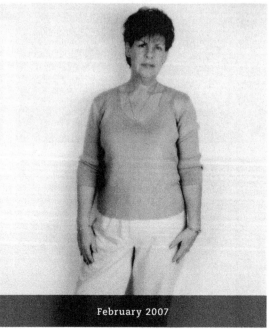

February 2007

bracelet—one that didn't stretch, but a solid band. Wearing a bracelet might have been a little thing, as things go, but to me it was a huge milestone. I wear it almost everyday as a reminder of just how far I've come.

By August, I was taken off my medications for high blood pressure, and plans were underway for the second wedding.

On September 1, the day of the second wedding, I celebrated not only the joys of welcoming the second of two treasured and beautiful daughters into the family, but I had lost 100 pounds.

Speaking of weddings, I was having a honeymoon of my own. Typically, these first six months are referred to as the *"honeymoon stage."* It is this physical recovery period right after surgery which holds the greatest window of opportunity for significant weight loss.

The weight just seems to melt away without much effort. Like most weight loss patients, at this point I was so thrilled I had the surgery. I was so enamored and in love with the realization of renewed health and so caught up in the bliss and excitement of rapid weight loss that the little bumps in the road don't seem to matter much. Compliments were pouring in and people everywhere were noticing my new figure.

During the Thanksgiving and Christmas holidays, I actually lost weight: 10 pounds. Yeah! I was wearing a size 14 W (Women's), but at least it wasn't an X size.

January 2007, my waist size was down from 47 inches to 32 inches.

On February 14, 2007, I was taken off my last prescription medication for thyroid. It was a huge emotional moment.

March marked a new size in clothing, a regular size 14. I could also get into a size 12. Although 12's were a little small, I purchased those, too. I could actually wear a regular size from Target and Talbots and could fit into small to medium shirts and sweaters.

In April, I celebrated my one-year surgery anniversary by reaching the first goal of weighing 170 pounds, which was the weight goal that the surgeon had set. I'd lost 132 pounds. I felt as though I was living a miracle.

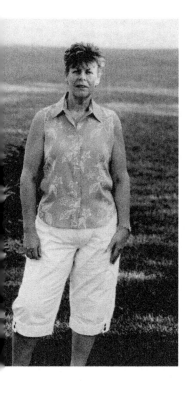

In April, I celebrated my one-year surgery anniversary by reaching the first goal of weighing 170 pounds

I wasn't done yet. Even though the weight loss started to slow, with diligent compliance to diet and exercise, this weight loss "window" can remain open for a while longer. Depending on the amount of weight one has to lose and the procedure chosen, this weight loss phase could last two years or more.

I set a new personal goal to comfortably fit into a size 12 and to be a little closer to the *normal* weight on the BMI chart.

Meanwhile, the Israelites witnessed many more miraculous encounters. As they made their way from the Red Sea, God continued to lead, guide, and provide for them. He turned bitter water into sweet. He led them to a nurturing and shady desert oasis of springs and palms. Even though it wasn't the paradise they were looking for just yet, it was a taste of what was to come. Well known for their fruitfulness, medicinal qualities, and longevity, the fruit from these palms provided sweet "honey" which is a symbol of healing, well-being, and provision. These were reminders that the land of promise was within their reach.

For me it seemed that way, too. Losing weight was a refreshing change from all the bitter years I had spent trying to lose weight unsuccessfully. Life was getting sweeter all the time. Remember the lap I wanted? I now had one. Just in time, too. Within a few months, I would be holding our first grandchild. What a year! What a life!

There were a lot of successes, but it wasn't easy street. Transitioning into a new way of life doesn't mean your troubles are over.

CHAPTER 20

Manna Matters and Buffet Blues

**When we are no longer able to change a situation,
we are challenged to change ourselves.**

Victor Frankl

It seemed as though things were going fine for the Israelites so long as there were no challenges, inconveniences, or discomforts. It wasn't too long (only a few weeks, actually) after the Red Sea miracle that things got a little difficult, and their rejoicing started to dissipate. They were out of Egypt but it didn't mean they were suddenly in the land of promise—they were in the desert.

Their Promised Land was only an eleven-day journey away. Once out of Egypt, they expected to be at or near their destination by now (a land flowing with "milk and honey", blessings and fruitfulness) They hadn't anticipated spending so much time in the middle of the desert.

Living life in the desert was a whole new experience. Although life in captivity was unbearably cruel, their former stay along the Nile was in a bustling and prosperous city filled with abundant resources. They were given food for their families and green pastures for their flocks and herds. In Egypt, they prospered and grew in number.

But there in the desert, things were different. There weren't sufficient supplies for this great multitude of people. They had to learn to trust in a different source to meet their needs. They had to learn to trust in God's personal care and provision.

As their thirst and hunger began to become more apparent, food started to take center stage. They started to complain and grumble about the lack of food.

God still continued to perform miracles. He gave them sweet tasting manna (or bread from heaven) that met all their nutritional needs everyday—breakfast, lunch, and dinner. Even though the manna was to be gathered under specific instructions and within measure, God supplied ample provisions to meet every individual need without fail and without toil. He supplied water from the rocks, and multiplied the number of quail for them to eat. As an added bonus, their clothes didn't wear out, and He kept them in good health. But still, they were not happy.

They began to dwell on what they *didn't* have, instead of what they *did*. Their losses seemed to outweigh the benefit they had gained. Instead of turning their focus to their newly-found freedom and health. They didn't just want to *return* to Egypt, they wished they had *died* in Egypt. *"If only we had died by the Lord's hand in Egypt. There we sat around pots of meat and ate all the food we wanted, but you have brought us out into this desert to starve this entire assembly to death." (Exodus 16:3)*

Is it me or does it seem to you that the memory of their former way of life in Egypt was getting a little warped by the searing heat of the desert? This wilderness can do that, you know. The truth about their way of life in Egypt shows signs of decline, distortion, and over-exaggeration. They recalled sitting around pots of meat and eating all they wanted. We have been told in scripture that they had entered Egypt with livestock, but some historians say that sitting around pots of meat and eating all they wanted was not a customary part of the life of slaves.

But even if they did enjoy the "all you can eat, anytime you want," buffets while in Egypt, they seem to be deceiving themselves into imagining a life of luxury—forgetting their former life was racked with misery, pain, turmoil, and impending death. Even so, it is doubtful that during the plagues, or while their infants were being drowned in the river, that they had even considered death as a practical alternative.

Remember, for us in the bariatric world, we are also experiencing a transition into a new life. During my recovery process there was more taking place than just physical healing from surgery and pinnacles of weight loss grandeur. My healthier choices were allowing me to assume better physical health, but then there was the aftermath of change.

Many of the changes taking place in my life were spectacular, but there were changes that weren't so thrilling. I was experiencing the fulfillment of promises of restoration, but as these physical transitions began to unfold, my relationship with food was starting to be significantly obvious. The bar on the scale may have been going in a downward direction, but as these emotional challenges begin to surface, the emotional bar began to rise. Feelings seemed to appear out of nowhere without warning. These weren't just momentary events. They became regular occurrences. I began to experience a few buffet blues of my own.

It's My Seafood And I'll Cry If I Want To

We were vacationing on the islands of the Outer Banks of North Carolina for a week with some friends. My husband, Richard, and I often eat dinner out, and we usually share a meal. I really don't mind, most of the time. But this was vacation. And being on vacation, I had the expectation that I should be able to eat exactly what I wanted—within my boundaries, of course. We had discussed our options. We planned to share a meal and agreed on what we would order: grilled seafood. But at the last minute, while ordering, he decided to switch to a selection of fried seafood—which I couldn't eat. So, not only did I have to rethink my selection but I also had to deal with the serge of emotions that followed.

I could have chosen the shrimp cocktail, but it was vacation and I could order that at restaurants at home. We live within a mile of the ocean, and fresh seafood is readily available. Where is the treat in cold shrimp? It's so ordinary and this is a special occasion. I don't get to eat at *this* restaurant every day, and *everybody* else got to order exactly what *they* wanted!

I don't mind being unique, but this kind of "different" didn't feel good. Most all of the selections I could eat were very expensive, so let's also add guilt to the list. I was at the point of tears.

Quietly, I excused myself from the table to find a place of solitude. Here it comes again, that pity-party moment. I could hear the music playing already, *It's My Party And I'll Cry If I Want To!*

You Should Cry Too, When It Happens to You

Food has been a good friend, support, comfort, and love for a long time. The quantity of food has changed as well as the type of food.

FIVE PHASES OF GRIEF.
Denial
Anger
Bargaining
Depression
Acceptance

Understanding the role food plays in our lives and identifying feeling over the loss of food is important as we make our way through this wilderness transition. Knowing that these feeling are a normal part of the process and why they occur is essential. In order to recover it is important to address them. These emotions offer us clues to determine where we are in the process, help us to recognize the core issues, and assist us in confronting them.

One of my close friends, La Cretia, was one of the indispensable cheerleaders on my support team. She understood what I was going through and helped me through this phase of emotional ups and downs.

She explained to me about the five phases of loss or grief. They may look similar to this:

- Denial (This isn't happening to me, or What have I done?)
- Anger (Why is this happening to me? I don't want to give up that food. I want to go back.)
- Bargaining (I promise I'll be a better person if; or I'll do better next time, it's only this once, or it's only a little)

- Depression (I don't care anymore;
  or experiencing self-pity)
- Acceptance (I'm ready for whatever comes.
  I'm going to succeed. I can do it.)

The first four stages in the process follow no prescribed order or length of duration and can be experienced over and over again. You may go through each of these stages or experience one phase more than another. *"So how do I stop it?"* I asked. Acceptance is the key.

Acceptance means to take or receive with approval, changing our thought process, adopting a new mindset, choosing to believe that things will be favorable, and trusting that life is not over.

I think it is important to know beforehand that these feelings are common and are experienced by most weight loss surgery patients. Passing through these phases is probably and regretfully inescapable. Knowing how to maneuver through them is indispensable. The most important thing is not to set up camp in these different stages of grief, but to accept the new reality, progress forward, and move on into the new way of life.

Choosing Acceptance

Our lives are a series of choices and we all hold the ability and the freedom to choose. As we walk along this path from pre-surgery into maintenance we will find plenty of opportunities in which to exercise this freedom. I thought by having gastric bypass surgery I was giving up my freedom to choose. I was wrong. I have plenty of choices. The question is, whether I use these choices to improve my health and my life or whether I choose to go back into the old way of living.

Even though we so desperately long to be free from the strangling appetites and emotions within, there is strong opposition that seems to pull us back. We imagine that going back would be easier than going forward. It may seem as though

I thought by having gastric bypass surgery I was giving up my freedom to choose. I was wrong.

we are not equipped to undergo such strong conflict. It may feel as though we have been abandoned on another one of life's battlefields. We can feel as if we have been "cheated" out of the best that life has to offer.

The place in which we find ourselves is not what we expected. It doesn't feel like home. It is neither comfortable nor pleasant. This unfamiliar territory can be disorienting and frightening. Our security has been breached and we feel exposed, insecure, and lost. We long to return to the familiar. We know we shouldn't but it seems extremely tempting and deceivingly unavoidable. We find ourselves at a crossroad with no obvious road-markers or directions.

- **Q** What now?
- **Q** Where do I go from here?
- **Q** How do I adjust?
- **Q** How do I deal with the emotional upheaval?
- **Q** How do I free myself from the things that threaten to rob me of my success?
- **Q** Where can I go for comfort?
- **Q** How do I acclimate to this new life?
- **Q** Where can I find a place of safety?
- **Q** Will I ever be happy in this new place?

That evening on the Outer Banks, I had to give myself a very strong pep talk in front of the restroom mirror. It was not about the seafood. It went much deeper than what I was eating. I had to confront "what was eating me." It was the realization that change had to come and I had to accept it. These emotional moments allowed me to confront the problem head on. It allowed me to recognize the areas in which I needed inward change and acceptance and turn them into victories. I had to come face-to-face with the real questions.

It's not that an occasional variance from the eating guideline is never allowed; it's about establishing a different mindset. I did have the power, right, and privilege to choose what I wanted.

Q   What do I want?

Q   What are the options?

Before surgery, I made a commitment toward a healthier life. I had to remind myself of my objectives. I had to review my commitment. I had to focus on refocusing. This and other similar moments brought me to realize that I had to change my perspective, to focus on what was important in life. This included retraining my thought process to include gratitude. I made an effort to reconnect with the positive aspects of what I was gaining in the process and focus on the benefits and rewards that this new life has to offer.

I have the option to remain enslaved and tangled in the web of addictive behaviors and emotional disorders or choose to face the changes, follow the path to freedom, and rid myself of these captors.

There will always be vacations, birthdays, weddings, and other occasions in which to sway from the new lifestyle. I must choose carefully and not fall back into old habits. This is when it helps to remember where I came from.

Q   Do I want to go back to the old?

Q   Am I willing to keep moving forward
        in the right direction?

Q   What choices will I make?

Self-entitlement comes with a lot of unsightly baggage. There is a difference between having the freedom to choose and making wise choices. Good or bad, I will pay the cost for what I want and what I choose.

Q   Will my choices be a wise and healthy?

Q   Will they be choices that will take me toward
        my goal or will they lead me into more defeat,
        depression, disease, heartache, or even death?

Q Will I use this crisis opportunity to grow toward spiritual maturity or remain in self-centeredness?

Choosing to have surgery comes with risk, but so does living life after surgery. My choices determined my direction, my path, and my future. Every day, every moment I have the opportunity to make a choice, to take a different course.

Learning how to accept these lifestyle changes had to become a priority for success. Once I make the choice to accept these changes with a positive mindset, positive feelings began to follow.

After pulling myself together that night, I returned to the table. Looking back, I don't remember what I ate for dinner. But what I do remember from that evening (beyond the emotional acceptance episode) was the great fellowship we shared with our friends as we watched the most gorgeous sunset over the sound.

I had pity-party moments for quite some time, but they came fewer and farther apart. Well, actually—the truth be told—I still have an occasional pity-party moment.

Having supporters in my life is invaluable for dealing with these emotional stages of recovery because it often feels as if you are going through it alone. I need emotional support for dealing with crisis moments as well as cheerleaders who keep me focused on the progress I have made. It helps tremendously to have lots of friends and family on my team and a great local support group, as well as dozens of weight loss patient friends who understand what I'm going through. There are even times I have to seek professional counseling and coaching.

In her book, *Balcony People*, Joyce Landorf Heatherley refers to these supporters as "balcony" people, those who are in our corner encouraging us on to success. These are people who "*love, listen, and care from the heart....affirmers who encourage you to stretch and dream beyond your self-imposed limits and capabilities.*"

Even though these supporters are incredibly important, I have also learned to be my own encourager. That night in the seafood restaurant, even though I was with family and friends, this personal internal struggle was something that I had to deal with on my own. I have to continually remind myself of the reason I made the decision to have surgery.

There are so many changes that come on this road to recovery, and the process takes time. In these transitional seasons, I find my journal is a huge help in rebuilding my hope and rekindling my desire to go forward.

I encourage you to face the challenges and the change. Expect these moments to come, be prepared before surgery and during the months that follow. Make moments of grief brief and allow opportunities for emotional healing and inward growth. The end result of these grief moments must always be the same, acceptance.

I have found that these emotional moments turn into huge milestones and give me an opportunity to experience tremendous emotional satisfaction and spiritual growth.

Yes, things are different, but they can also be better. Once you accept the loss, you are on your way to recovery and a new outlook on life. After surgery, you can still enjoy food, the social experience, and learn to enjoy life more. The best is yet to be.

Out of Obesity by Julia Holloman

CHAPTER 21

New Land, New Rules, New Purpose

**You have brains in your head. You have feet in your shoes.
You can steer yourself any direction you choose.
You're on your own. And you know what you know.
And YOU are the one who'll decide where to go.**

Dr. Seuss

The Israelites may have been mourning the loss of the "all you can eat buffets" that they had left behind in Egypt, but God was preparing them for the ultimate upgrade. As promised, God had faithfully delivered them out of bondage. He led them through the desert to Mount Sinai where He positioned them for success.

This spectacular mountain view came complete with front row seats in which they were given an opportunity to see the keynote speaker up close and personal—God Himself. As the discourse commences, He told the Israelites that He would establish them as a valuable and treasured nation. Assured that the land belonged to them, they were told of the riches and the many incredible blessings that awaited their arrival.

In order to enjoy exclusive lifetime access to the Promised Land, all they had to do was follow a few rules. He gave them important information about what life would be like from that point on and how they could prosper in the new land. Once inside their new territory, God would establish their borders and boundaries. There would be enemies and obstacles, but God assured them they could be overcome. His plan was to send angels to guard and protect them along the way. He encouraged them to be strong and courageous and to go in and take possession of the land. He promised to bless them, bless their food and water, take away sickness, keep them free from disease, make them fruitful, and to give them a full life.

However, none of these things would happen by their efforts alone, and it would not be an immediate event. These promises were conditional. In return, the Israelites had to completely demolish the enemies that ruled the land, trust God, and follow Him wholeheartedly.

Moving to A Higher Place

God introduced, what we refer to as the Ten Commandments. For the Israelites, these words offered them an ideal model for success. Their compliance to these guidelines would enhance their lives, ensure their freedom, allow them to build a strong new nation, and permit them to prosper in their newfound freedom.

We, too, must comply with a few guiding principles in order to build a strong new body and enjoy healing, health, and long life. By following the protocols of our new land, we position ourselves to move toward the Promised Land.

The Ten Commandments for Weight Loss Surgery Success

I.   Choose compliance with all thy heart.
II.   Thou shalt remember thy eating and keep it healthy.
III.   Thou shalt observe thy new behaviors
       until they become habits.
IV.   That shalt take care of thy new body.
V.   Honor thy new (altered) reality.
VI.   Thou shalt establish a new way of thinking.
VII.   Thou shalt no longer use false labels
       and negative self-talk.
VIII. Thou shalt remember thy past, but not dwell there.

IX.   Thou shalt align thy expectations and thy
      relationships according to thy new likeness.
X.   Thou shalt not be ruled by weight
      regain, fear, or other masters.

Just as in the biblical commandments, these standards are divided into two groups. There are physical and social elements, (practical tools and procedures for everyday living) and there are mental, emotional, and spiritual boundaries, (a new way of thinking that will allow the old habits and old ways of thinking to be torn down and allow new ones to be established.)

It will become extremely important to take care of our new body. We will need new foods to feed our body, new eating habits for our altered anatomy, and adjustments in our activity level. But as we transition into our new land, our success will require more than just rules that pertain to what we eat and how much we exercise. Taking care of our new body will require us to make other lifestyle choices as well.

For those of us who seek to gain improved health and to reach, as well as maintain weight loss surgery success, we must learn how to feed our body, soul, and spirit. These guidelines allow us to become stronger emotionally, mentally, and spiritually. In addition, they will help us rebuild our self-image, establish stronger relationships, discover new things about our ability to be compliant, and realize our spiritual identity.

Our priority, from this point on, will require our willingness to make these changes and follow the guidelines for success.

Please note that after surgery, you will most likely receive a list of guidelines, or suggestions, as well as hard fast rules for taking care of your altered anatomy. Let's take a look at these post-surgical guidelines as well as the rules. I'll also share other things I found helpful, what life was like for me, and how I made these adjustments as I made my way out of obesity and onward into my Promised Land.

Out of Obesity by Julia Holloman

CHAPTER 22

I. Choose Compliance With All Thy Heart

Our bodies are our gardens - our wills are our gardeners.
William Shakespeare

I, too, found that life held a renewed sense of purpose. Our family was given one of the biggest little gifts life has to offer. We welcomed the priceless wonder of our first grandchild, a little boy named Gavin, into our lives. My new lap has given me plenty of invaluable and indescribable pleasures of holding this little guy next to my heart, right where he belongs.

But even in the midst of all of life's wonderful celebrations, things don't always go as planned. There were still challenges—unsuspected temptations that sought to draw me back to the past and undermine my best intentions to be compliant.

I found myself standing in front of leftover birthday cake. I was just going to have a little sliver, one tiny little taste. Then one led to another and another. Just one more, a tiny little piece. You know, just to even out the edges. No one will ever miss it. After all, it was just cake. I wasn't eating all the icing.

As I stood there whittling away, an old familiar image began to come into focus. There she was, as clear as day. I had opened the door and she was making herself right at home. Her 300-pound weight didn't slow the speed at which she entered the scene. A reflection of my former self, this was the girl I used to be. I thought I had dismissed her long ago. It stopped me in my tracks.

Hadn't I been a slave to those old out-of-control feelings long enough? How long would I allow this cunning enemy to rob me of my hard earned success, my future, and my life? Was it delivering what it promised? It was another moment of decision. At this moment I could choose to continue to give in to its power, or I could choose to break free of its vice-like grip.

Disguised as creamy white frosting with multi-colored sprinkles, it had subtly enticed me with sugary promises, and I had believed it. I was shocked that something as flimsy as yellow cake held such power over me. As I stood there face-to-face, I realized I didn't want to be that person anymore. I promptly announced that she was no longer welcome as I shoved all of the half-eaten leftover cake into the trash.

Footstools and Kisses

Egyptian Pharaohs were the rulers of one of the greatest kingdoms of the ancient world, and to the people of Egypt, they were a god. Not only did the pharaohs of Egypt rule the land of Egypt and the great kingdoms along the river Nile, their power and influence reached to places far beyond their homeland as they sought to conquer and rule other territories, as well. There were also more enemies in addition the ones in Egypt who sought to regain control, plenty more waited ahead for an opportunity to confront them.

We may find, also, that just because we have won the battles of the past, doesn't mean the war is over just yet.

It brought to mind another biblical story in the book of *I Kings* as King Solomon prepared to build the temple. He recounts that before the temple could be built, all the enemies had to be overcome. He must have total dominion over his kingdom, and peace must rule the land.

The metaphor used here is, *"making his enemies a footstool."* The footstool was fastened to the throne in those days, and having his enemies under his feet communicated his authority and victory over them.

Solomon's father, David, had dealt with the national enemies of the kingdom, but Solomon encountered internal challenges—those close to him who sought to take over the throne.

Weight loss surgery offers us help in managing our outward or physical foes by reducing the size of our stomachs; in turn helping us establish healthy boundaries and proper portion control. It gives us the opportunity to regain control of our physical kingdom. But beware, this time will be short-lived, and there are old internal enemies that will come calling again. The job of maintaining these new boundaries and uprooting these internal foes is left up to us.

I had to do some soul-searching to discover what I really wanted. When I stand face-to-face with temptation, will I stand for freedom or captivity? Am I willing to fight for freedom?

I first realized I didn't like the person I was stuffing cake into my mouth. That was a big step. I had to learn how to stand my ground and exercise my right to choose. I chose to let go of those old habits. I chose to believe I was not the same person I had been before. I chose not to be that girl anymore. I refused to let cake control me and take away the territory I had worked so hard to conquer.

I'm not going to say the girl I used to be might not come knocking at the door again; but next time she threatens, she will find a stronger guard there. After that moment, I had a stronger resolve to stand watch over the entry points and make sure she knew she was not free to take up residence.

These internal adversaries may be different for each one of us, but we all face them. They can be overcome, and they must, in order for us to build our new life in a land ruled by peace and harmony. We can resume control of those out-of-control moments. We must be willing and determined to identify these old habits and not allow unwanted behaviors to succeed in their attempt to rule us. It is important to be willing to be compliant to the guidelines and to make a choice to be free from the things that hold us in the past—wholeheartedly.

We have a new territory to defend, and we have paid a great price to achieve it. Easy? No. I have to work at establishing my footstool. There are still battles left to fight.

Possible? Yes. It may take some effort to uproot those intruders, but we can do it.

This is the reason I had surgery: life, and to live life to the fullest.

As I recorded that moment in my journal, a few weeks later, I flipped through the photos of Gavin's birthday. Our daughter, Millie, had taken a photo of Gavin and me. I am sitting on the back porch on a footstool and he is sitting in my lap, an appropriate image for me.

This is the reason I had surgery: life, and to live life to the fullest. This is part of the territory I'm willing to lay my life down to defend. A future that holds the promise of greater health in which to see this little one grow, and all those who come after. Establishing memories of running in the yard, playing hide and seek, blowing and chasing bubbles. I couldn't do that before. Moments like these have given me many grand occasions for this little one to sit in my lap, and I can get all the kisses and hugs my heart desires. These moments are sweeter than any cake.

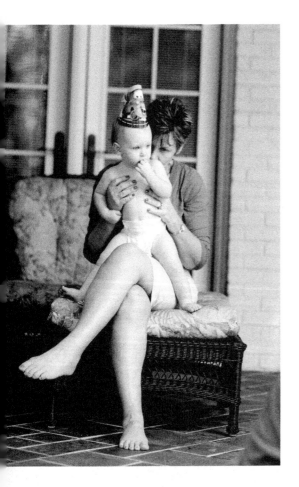

Life goes on. It brings with it the greatest pleasures of inward growth and opportunities, not only of enjoyment, but of leaving a future legacy to the next generations to come. It's great to be alive, and it's great to be a MeMe. I'm learning to put those enemies under my feet. You, too, can celebrate the victories of your footstool moments.

CHAPTER 23

II. Thou Shalt Remember Thy Eating and Keep It Healthy

Oh, my friend, it's not what they take away from you that counts. It's what you do with what you have left.

Hubert Humphrey

During our journey, we will move through several transitional food phases from clear liquids, full liquids, and soft foods before we can resume a regular food diet. But our "normal" will not be the same as it was before surgery. As we transition through these food phases, there will be guidelines and countless opportunities to practice compliance—to eat, drink, and chew well.

These were the guiding principles I followed from the beginning of my weight loss phase and they still remain a part of my daily plan.

Eat Well

Eating well means choosing well. Once on a regular diet, it is wise to choose a wide variety of healthy, colorful, and whole foods that are as close to nature as possible. After surgery, eating for health and proper nutrition must become a priority. Eating healthy will determine the difference between having good health or poor health.

Protein will become one of those new priorities. Eat protein first and always.

Balanced eating will include eating healthy fats, such as nuts and seeds, olives, olive oil, other plant oils such as avocados, and yes, even dark chocolate. Your body needs fat. Fat delivers nutrients to your body. Fat slows down digestion. It is also heavy on the stomach. Eating too much can make you feel as though you swallowed a brick. Eating too much fat may also cause dumping. (We will discuss "dumping" in an upcoming chapter.)

It will also be important to choose healthy carbohydrates such as fruits, green and starchy vegetables, whole grains, sweet potatoes, and quinoa. We must avoid highly processed foods (except on occasion). Carbohydrates are not "bad" foods, and it doesn't call for total elimination, but it does involve making wise choices and remaining within our bariatric portion sizes.

Eat on Purpose

It is important not to skip meals or overeat. Eat enough not to be hungry later. Eating small meals frequently increases calorie burn and speeds up your metabolism. Our metabolism is affected by several things:

- Nutrition - the type, frequency, and amount of food eaten
- Hydration - the amount of water we drink
- Physical activity – how much we exert ourselves
- Bone structure, body type, genetic make-up, and body composition (that is, the amount of muscle we have compared to the amount of fat)
- Properly functioning organs, glands, and hormones

Eating protein, for example, increases your metabolism by up to 30 percent and fiber around 15 percent. Meals have the potential to boost our metabolic rate up to two hours after we eat.

Remember, after weight loss surgery, we will be eating less food per meal than before surgery. Eat several smaller, well-balanced meals, including in-between mini-meals or snacks. Small meals and snacks should be balanced and healthy, not continual grazing. When your portions are small, you should eat every 2 to 3 hours (or no longer than 4) to maintain strength and avoid "ups and downs" in blood sugar. These meals and in-between mini-meals should consist of complex carbohydrates balanced with protein.

The purpose of eating is nourishment, keeping your body energized, strong, and balanced. Eating for health and, yes, pleasure. Choose wisely and enjoy eating in moderation. Observe the variety of unique colors, tastes, textures, and aromas. When you are done, you should be satisfied not shameful.

The 5, 10, 15 Guideline

After surgery, I was given a guideline—which was nick-named the 5, 10, 15 rule. I have found that staying within the 5, 10, 15, boundaries has been a great way to maintain health, prevent dumping, keep losing weight, prevent significant weight regain, and regulate low blood sugar levels.

The 5, 10, 15, is actually a flexible *guideline*, not a hard-fast rule. The idea is to limit your fat to 5 grams per meal or within single digits. Sugar should be limited to 10 grams or less per meal. Carbs should be around 15 to 20 grams per meal. Eating food high in sugar and carbs may cause dumping.

Everybody is different. Eating after surgery requires a little time to experiment with what works for you. It will require that you be diligent in finding your own limits for weight loss and keeping your body at the weight you want.

Although lap-band and gastric bypass guidelines may differ, the 5, 10, 15, guideline is a good overall plan that's easy to remember. It is also a good guide for those trying to lose weight without surgery, as well. I found this easy to follow. I have followed this guide since the beginning of my weight loss phase and have continued to do so on into maintenance.

Know Your Portions

Keep in mind that there is a difference between a *portion* and a *serving*.

A *serving* size is a certain standard measure or quantity of food by weight or volume. Package listing will tell you the *serving* size used to calculate certain nutritional counts.

A *portion* is dependent upon the amount of food one *chooses* to eat. A bariatric portion is smaller than the standard for normal folks, especially in the beginning months.

In the beginning my portion *size* (or amount of food I was allotted), was determined by my food phase, (e.g. ¼ cup or ½ cup). While in the clear liquid, full liquid, and soft food phases, my limit was ½ cup portions per meal.

When I entered the regular food phase, my limits changed from no less than ½ cup and no more than a cup per meal. The food I selected also had to fit within the principles of the 5, 10, 15 guideline.

In order to calculate my *personal portion*, or bariatric friendly size, I used the *standard serving size* and adjusted the amounts accordingly to correspond to my food phase.

Let's say I wanted to eat a sweet potato. A sweet potato is a nutritious whole food vegetable, and would be considered a healthy choice. Sweet potatoes contain carbohydrates. My bariatric guideline is between 15 and 20 grams of carbohydrates per meal. My new bariatric portion size would be between 1/3 cup (which contains approximately 14 grams of carbs) and a ½ cup (which contains approximately 21 grams of carbs). Any other carbohydrate I choose to eat for that particular meal must also be calculated. But my guideline for carbohydrates for that meal is between 15 and 20 grams.

Your bariatric portion is dependent on your guideline for weight loss, maintenance, health, and other dietary boundaries after surgery. Remember, this is a guide to help you know the healthier food-item choices.

Does this mean you can never eat dessert again? No. Not necessarily. After the weight loss phase, I learned how to

> A *serving* size is a certain standard measure or quantity of food by weight or volume.

> A *portion* is dependent upon the amount of food one *chooses* to eat.

manage small bites and still accomplish my goal for better health. For example: dark chocolate is heart healthy (as long as it doesn't trigger food sensitivities or addictions). I limit my chocolate choice to dark, very little sugar, the highest cocoa content possible, and small portions.

I recommend not adding desserts back into your diet until you have completed the weight loss phase and are confident that you can remain in control. Even now, there are still food items I struggle to keep within the limits, so I avoid those food items. I have to set my personal boundaries.

Remember the idea is to make wise, whole food choices that provide our body with good nutrition. Adding high calorie foods, refined sugars, highly processed, or non-nutritive foods should be done sparingly and within the bounds of caution.

I suggest you be mindful that the foods you eat are within your timeline of food phases that you are allowed during the healing and weight loss process for your safety and health. Again, these are suggested guidelines. Everyone is different and must find what works for individual success.

I recommend you follow the guidelines of your surgeon or dietitian first and foremost, if you are given any.

Learning how to make healthier food choices must become permanent and will accompany smaller portion sizes for the long-term.

Smaller Plate, Smaller Portions

There are two helpful habits I have discovered to avoid overeating—using a smaller plate and measuring my portions. Studies show that we are usually conditioned to eat the amount on our plate and we tend to find ourselves satisfied, regardless of portion size. I have found this to be true.

Using a smaller plate has been useful. In time, the plate and the amount of food I put on it, became my new normal. No matter where I am, a restaurant or private home, I usually ask for a small plate.

> Learning how to make healthier food choices must become permanent and will accompany smaller portion sizes for the long-term.

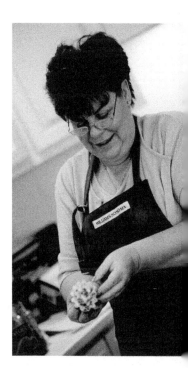

Measuring Success

Along with making wiser food choices, comes practicing new routines of measuring new food portion sizes. Measuring cups, spoons, and a food scale are excellent tools which work together to help your new pouch *tool* remain small.

In the beginning we start with drinking ½ cup meal portions. Then we move to eating ½ cup meal portions—equally divided into protein and carbohydrates.

The portion sizes we can eat increases as time goes on. Within a year we may be able to eat a cup of food. For the long-term, our guideline will be no less than ½ cup and no more than a cup.

Remember, the 5, 10, 15 guideline serves as the new standard for portions. I found it extremely important to measure my new portion sizes on a regular basis until my mind's eye could recall the difference in each measured portion such as 1/4 or 1/3 of a cup of food, without using the measuring cup.

A protein serving size for normal folks is 3 to 4 ounce or a *card size* portion. But after weight loss surgery, my new protein portion is 2 to 3 ounces. Memorizing these new portion sizes helped me establish my new way of eating. It was helpful to memorize portion sizes for the long-term.

Using a size reference, such as a deck of cards or a ping pong ball, for each food group portion is especially valuable for those times when measuring is not convenient. In the beginning, I always measured everything I ate or drank. During the journey, I still take a moment from time to time to make sure my guesses are still correct.

Drink Well

Getting enough fluids is an important consideration after surgery. Sipping fluids will be necessary in the days ahead to avoid dehydration. For new weight loss surgery patients, getting enough liquids may be challenging because you will only be taking in a few teaspoons at a time. But keep trying. This amount will increase as time goes on.

Skip the straw! Drinking from a straw will cause air in the stomach, which will be very painful.

So why is it so important to drink (or sip, in our case) so much fluid? We all know hydration is important, but did you know drinking water helps you lose weight and have healthier skin?

Your liver plays a huge role in detoxification and burning fat. Your kidneys flush out the fat and toxins from your body. But when you don't drink enough fluids your liver has to work harder to detoxify your system, so your liver can't burn as much fat as it could. Drinking water also helps your skin stay healthy and after all that weight loss, healthy and supple skin is important, too. So when you drink enough fluids you are helping your body help you lose weight, get healthy, and look great.

Remember, your protein shake can be included into your liquid count. You may find adding lemon, lime, orange, or even cucumber slices are refreshing additions to low calorie beverages.

Carbonated beverages do not offer sufficient hydration and can cause dehydration. They are very acidic and can negatively affect the new pouch. Carbonation causes gas bubbles, which stretches your small pouch, (and the opening leading from the stomach to the intestines), causing pain and compromising your new weight loss tool. These are best eliminated from your diet.

Tea is a good alternative, lower in caffeine, it offers as much hydration as water, and has loads of antioxidants to help you return to health.

Lap-band patients may find drinking warm liquids (especially in the morning) relaxes tight tummy muscles. So drink for your health.

Remember alcoholic beverages may not be a good choice after weight loss surgery and are best avoided. Alcohol is more rapidly absorbed after mal-absorptive surgery. It contains higher acidity level, which can result in ulcers, and high amounts of sugar, which causes dumping. Alcohol can be addicting and can also lead to transfer addiction. (More about transfer addiction later)

The 30, 30, 30 Rule

Don't drink liquids while eating. This was perhaps the hardest one for me, over time it has become much easier. The new limit is 30, 30, 30. No drinking 30 minutes before eating, 30 minutes during the meal, and at least 30 minutes after eating.

It's not that you can't have something handy in case you need to take a little sip. The idea is that liquids not only wash food from your pouch, but liquids also fill your pouch, resulting in less food eaten, leaving you hungry again. Since portion sizes are small, nutrition is especially important. Liquids also dilute digestive juices that you need. Remember your stomach doesn't work the same as it used to. This is when chewing becomes important by helping things go down smoother.

Chew Well

Chewing well requires an element of concentration. You will want to make it a habit for the long-term. Your stomach no longer churns and mixes like it did before. Your digestive juices are not at the maximum, so chewing assists in the digestion process and will help relieve the need to drink while eating.

Chewing well also prevents foods from getting stuck in the opening of your new pouch, which is a serious complication that will require medical attention. Chew your food until it is the consistency of applesauce before swallowing.

While we are on the subject of chewing, there is one thing that you don't want to chew—chewing gum. Just as with a straw, chewing gum allows air in the stomach, which causes pain.

Slow Down and Be Mindful

Don't eat in a hurry. Eating should take about 20 to 30 minutes, not 5. Eat sitting down—not in the car, standing, or on the run.

Use small eating utensils, even chop sticks.

Be mindful. Stay alert and focused. Mealtime is a great opportunity to relax, refocus from the thoughts of the day to enjoy the meal. You may soon discover that mindful eating is a weight loss surgery patient's best friend.

Take small bites. I suggest putting down your fork between each bite. Concentrate on the taste and texture of the food.

Limit distractions. When listening or engaging in conversation, I find it helpful to put my fork down and concentrate on the conversation. It's sometimes hard to pay attention to the food going into my mouth when there is a lot going on around me. This is why it's so important to have only the food you plan on eating on your plate. This was especially helpful early in the process.

All of these things are important and they take time to establish. Let's find out how to establish new habits.

CHAPTER 24

III. Thou Shalt Observe Thy New Behaviors Until They Become Habits

Self is the only prison that can ever bind the soul.

Henry Van Dyke

All these new changes will stretch us physically and emotionally. Meanwhile, our small pouch will be stretching its way though the healing process, too. It will help to understand how this process works.

Although there may be subtle differences in the way procedures are performed, or vary from surgeon to surgeon, RNY surgery is defined as a Y-shaped surgical connection that divides the small intestine to form two arms. One end of the small intestine (the jejunum) is attached to a *stoma* into a gastric pouch. The opposite end (the bypassed duodenum, which is the first part of the small intestine immediately beyond the stomach, leading to the jejunum, connects with an end-to-side anastomosis into the lower jejunum.

This procedure, known as gastric bypass surgery, reduces the size of the stomach over 90 percent. Your former *"normal"* stomach could stretch, sometimes to over 1000 ml (or four cups). The newly-formed pouch after gastric bypass is altered to be around 10 to 13 ml in size (or 1 tablespoon).

The gastric bypass pouch is usually formed from the part of the stomach that is the least susceptible to stretching. This, in addition to its small size, prevents any significant long-term change in pouch volume, *but the size of your pouch does stretch.* But this isn't the only change.

There is a valve, called a pyloric sphincter, between our "old" stomach and our small intestine. This valve controls the flow of digested food leaving the stomach. However, this valve is no longer a part of the new operating stomach pouch, which is created during the RNY procedure. Without this valve, food empties more quickly from the new pouch into the intestinal track. After surgery the size of this connection between the stomach and bowel is determined by the healing process, which controls the degree of tightness. If it is too tight, food cannot leave the pouch causing a stricture.

Over time, the size of the connection changes and stretches, as does the ability of the small bowel to hold a greater volume of food. These changes allow food to exit the stomach even more quickly. This is a natural part of the process.

Typically around the end of the first year, gastric bypass patients will be able to eat a greater quantity of food. This is also a time when hunger makes its return, genuine stomach hunger, as well as that dreaded head or emotional hunger. And, like it or not, (or even admit it to ourselves or not), old habits start to reappear. This is why understanding our changing anatomy and establishing new lifestyle habits are so crucially important to long-term success.

Did I Do That?

Before having weight loss surgery, one of my Saturday morning treats included going out to breakfast with my husband. After surgery, it has become mostly breakfast at home.

But this day, I was in the mood for an omelet. So when my husband announced he was taking me out to eat breakfast, I was excited.

So, off we went. I ordered the egg and cheese omelet with whole-wheat toast. As usual, when the food arrived, it was more than I could eat. I proceeded to divide the omelet in a bariatric friendly portion and placed all but one slice of the whole wheat toast onto another plate.

Covering half the plate was a huge mound of hash brown potatoes, which I had forgotten to tell them to leave off. I had chosen to spend my carbohydrate allotment on the toast. But before I could scoop them onto another plate (and unbeknownst to me) my right hand proceeded to squirt a half bottle of ketchup on those babies, and my fork was ready for the kill. Wait a minute! What was I doing? I didn't plan to eat the hash browns. And what was with all that ketchup? What was I thinking?

It seems I wasn't thinking at all, at least not about the present. My mind was somewhere else.

Why, at this point, did I empty an endless supply of ketchup onto a mountain-sized plateful of hash brown potatoes that I didn't plan to eat?

Habit. It's referred to in the bariatric world as *mindless eating*. This little habit was *"playin' possum"* as we say here in the South. The habit was pretending to be dead, in hopes that I would think it's no longer an issue. It was just waiting until I was unfocused and off guard to sneak up and attack. And it almost worked.

Did I do that? I was surprised and astounded! I really thought that habit was behind me and that my eating habits had forever changed. Not so, apparently.

That's just my point. You can never let your guard down. You know the verse, *"pride cometh before destruction and a haughty attitude before a fall."* Someone call the meek-squad! Ok, you possum-sized habit, you! You and your pride friend have been uncovered!

It is important to be focused and mindful when in the presence of food lest you find yourself saying likewise, *"Did I do that?"* Old habits die hard. Don't think it's over; it's not. Don't fool yourself into thinking those old habits are dead and gone. They may be just *"playin' possum,"* and when you least expect it, you could be caught red-handed with a bottle of ketchup.

Times like these are when it will be necessary to make a plan of success. I had to give my husband a heads-up on keeping me attentive. I needed to let him know that he had my permission to call me on any questionable behavior. I had to practice keeping my mind on what I was doing at mealtime and remember that no matter how long I'd been practicing good habits there was always a chance of a slip-up.

I Think My Self is in My Way

I pulled out a book I had read seven years earlier. I turned to a chapter on habits. In the page margin I had written the statement, *"My problem is not food; it is self!"* Yep! Self. And even here, even after weight loss surgery, the problem remained the same. Food was not the problem. It was my behavior. I am the one who has to make the deliberate decision to remain in control and not give in to negative habits. It doesn't happen overnight, nor is it easy.

Establishing new habits requires self-control, discipline, constant repetition, consistency, and time. Establishing these post-surgery habits early during those first few months after surgery is highly recommended. As we continue to repeat these new disciplines, over time positive new habits and behaviors will develop. I had to begin to retrain my brain to operate under new muscle memory until it became automatic.

Studies show that it takes around 800 times before our brain can recall or memorize new habits. Some say this muscle memory takes much longer and can take up to 10,000 repetitions before our brain activity can cultivate, process, and become routine.

It takes much more discipline than going on a diet, that you can quit any time you wish. In the beginning, our weight loss surgery tool of a small pouch *temporarily* curbs our appetites and forces us to eat smaller portions. This allows us the time to develop the disciplines we need in an environment that *temporarily* helps to enforce the decisions we make. As we establish new boundaries and practice these new basic steps and lifestyle skills, these new disciplines will be formed from within.

Over time, the weight comes off, but at the same time, our boundaries widen. Remember, you will be able to eat a greater quantity of food and experience the return of physical and emotional hungers. Notice, these surgery benefits are not permanent, the key word here is *temporarily*.

When we overeat, we stretch our stomach pouch beyond the intended boundary, compromising our new tool. If lifestyle changes aren't made and internalized, negative habits will bring us back again to the place where the problem started—inside ourselves. Therefore, for weight loss surgery to be successful long-term, it will be necessary to make the changes that establish new habits for the long-term.

For me, it's been helpful to remember the benefits success affords. This is when I rely on those goals I had written down earlier. I have to remind myself in moments of weakness why I had surgery in the first place. I have to ask myself:

We will get the end result we want when our desire to succeed is strong enough to make the necessary changes to overcome our negative habits and replace them with new positive habits.

Q What is my objective?

Q Is my desire to possess my goal stronger than the negative habit?

Q Am I willing to comply with the positive disciplines that are required in order to reach success?

Q Have I identified my unwanted habits?

Q Have I made the necessary lifestyle changes?

Q Have I developed a plan and strategy that will help me remain faithful to my new habits?

Q What internal convictions hold me to my commitment?

It all starts with the decisions we make. We will get the end result we want when our desire to succeed is strong enough to make the necessary changes to overcome our negative habits and replace them with new positive habits.

I was reminded again of my friend Hannah. She shared, "*I had a habit of watching TV and eating. So, instead of eating while watching TV, I had to make an intentional effort to keep my hands busy. I would paint my nails. I even tried knitting. There were times, though, that I had to just turn the TV off all together. I started reading more, which I really enjoy. It's hard to eat and read at the same time.*"

Hannah further realized how important changing her habits were when her 8-year-old son, John Michael, also started to notice that his desire to eat was triggered by TV commercials about food, even when he wasn't hungry. Hannah is not only retraining her own habits but instilling values that will be carried on to the next generation. Way to go, John Michael. Way to go, Hannah!

Gaining Ground

Most likely, at this point, you are overwhelmed. You are probably asking yourself, *"How in the world will I ever get the hang of it?"*

Remember when you first started driving a car and what the experience felt like? There were so many things to think about. There was so much to learn; giving proper turn signals, knowing how much tension to apply to the brake, learning how much pressure it took to accelerate the car smoothly and without jerks.

Then there was balancing your attention between keeping the car between the lines and knowing how to glance into the rear view mirror, the two side mirrors from left to right, observing the speed changes and limits, school zones, and railroad crossings, routine checks of the speedometer, the traffic going in all directions, intersections, and hundreds of road signs. Who can do all that?

You might have learned on a car that had gears to shift, which added a whole new dimension and required some fancy footwork. And if that weren't enough you had to learn among the plethora of details, how to make a three point turn, park on a hill, and parallel park. Was that scary or what?

We had to learn to drive not only offensively but also defensively. We had to learn how to drive under different weather conditions, the darkness of night, and during rush hour traffic. Then there was a written test, signs to remember, eye tests, not to mention the intimidating driving test. There were plenty of opportunities for parental correction and peer pressure, including those daunting blue lights threatening to pounce on our every mistake.

We most likely didn't start out perfect, either. While we were learning we had an experienced driver beside us. At first, we began with an instructor and a vehicle equipped with an emergency brake. Then we progressed to a licensed driver, and before long we progressed to a learner's permit and then on to get our permanent license.

Then there was learning to change a tire and the oil. When you became a car owner there were the responsibilities of car care, car insurance, and license renewals. Then there is regular maintenance such as tires, gas fill-ups, inspections, fluid checks, and engine checks. And don't forget those Saturday morning car washes for keeping up outside appearances.

When I became a parent, my children were introduced not only to the "normal" set of rules of the road, but I gave them my own set of rules. I did not allow my young teenagers to listen to music, receive or place phone calls, or have other passengers in the car until they had become more experienced drivers.

Like all those who are first learning how to drive, the more driving we did, the more experienced we became, and with experience came confidence. With the passing of time those little distractions weren't as likely to turn our attention from the main purpose, which was to arrive safely at our intended destination. As our driving skills progressed—more privileges were added and the restrictions lessened.

Even with all those things to juggle and things to learn, we learned it quite well. We were teenagers. We were tenacious, ambitious, resolute, persistent, and determined to be successful. We were unstoppable and invincible. Never once did we consider giving up. It never entered our mind that these new skills *could not or would not* be conquered. This new and exciting experience was one that held a promise of great rewards—the promise of new freedoms.

Just like learning to drive, the more consistent we become with our new eating habits, the sooner new ones will develop.

With time and practice, we will gain more wisdom in knowing how to steer clear of obstacles. Over time, these new habits will become easier and they won't consume our undivided attention. The more skilled we become, the further we can travel down the road to success. And once again we can look forward to the promise of new freedoms.

CHAPTER 25

IV. Thou Shalt Take Care
of Thy New Body

"When things go wrong, don't go with them."

Elvis Presley

Most people who have had weight loss surgery will tell you it is one of the best things they have ever done, even those who have faced unanticipated circumstances ranging from a few little bumps in the road to major complications.

We have discussed acceptance to diet, but there are other changes we need to consider.

These include physical changes as a *result* of weight loss surgery, important medical information, and lifestyle changes that will be necessary for success.

There are experiences that are specifically unique to bariatric patients, even though our bodies will respond differently to each surgical procedure.

Weight loss surgery demands that we start taking care of ourselves now more than ever.

For women, nurturing comes naturally, and we find ourselves nurturing others far more than ourselves. We have even come to think that time spent on ourselves is selfish.

Men often lean towards finding their identity and fulfillment in professions and careers. When things tend to go wayward it is a tendency to go with them, which allows these events to dictate self-value, importance, and purpose.

A lot of us don't view ourselves as important or valuable, but we are very valuable. We may have experienced some failure in one aspect of our lives, but we are not a failure. It's time we start to take the time to refresh and nurture ourselves.

It is important to take care of our physical body. Taking care of ourselves isn't selfish. It's no different than taking care of our basic physical needs. It's time we take care of our new body. It starts with understanding the importance of our new altered anatomy.

> It's time we take care of our new body. It starts with understanding the importance of our new altered anatomy.

Restriction and Mal-absorption

Most weight loss surgery procedures involve restriction, which alters the amount of food one can eat. Some procedures, such as gastric bypass, involve mal-absorption. Mal-absorption procedures alter the normal way the body breaks down fats, proteins, and carbohydrates one eats into smaller particles that the body can absorb. Although mal-absorption procedures cause a rapid amount of weight loss that tends to last longer than restrictive types alone, these options put one at a higher risk for long-term complications.

In order to achieve and maintain good health long-term, it is important to understand the need for new medical requirements. This helps us to avoid nutritional and vitamin deficiencies as well as other health related risks. With proper adjustments, these can be managed, but they will be with you for the rest of your life.

Early Dumping Syndrome

After returning to a regular food diet, we suffer consequences for making wrong food choices. However, most consequences can be avoided by following the guidelines.

All the side effects that surgery may have on the body overall or for the long term are not yet known. But there is one thing that is known and that is the consequence that happens when eating too much sugar. It is referred to as *dumping syndrome*.

Dumping syndrome is the direct result of alterations in the storage function of the stomach and/or the emptying mechanism. It is caused by the rapid entry of undigested foods, sugar, active solids, and liquids as they bypass absorption in the small intestine and "dump" directly into the duodenum—producing decreased blood pressure and increased blood flow to the intestines, causing severe cramps and uncontrollable diarrhea.

Early dumping occurs during the first year or two after surgery and usually within 15 to 30 minutes of eating foods high in sugar or fat.

Early dumping syndrome leads to generalized weakness. It will include, abdominal cramps, explosive diarrhea, and sweating. It may also include vomiting, fainting, irregular or rapid heartbeat, dizziness low blood pressure, flushing of the skin, and shortness of breath.

Dumping will be painful, disruptive, and very unpleasant, to say the least. You will want to avoid it at all cost. By avoiding refined sugars and remaining within the carbohydrate, sugar, and fat guidelines you are given by your surgeon, you can prevent dumping syndrome.

Alcohol is more rapidly absorbed after mal-absorptive surgery. Because it contains sugar, and creates a higher acidity level, it can result in ulcers as well as dumping. So, alcohol is best avoided.

These and other food sensitivities after surgery are different for everyone.

Vitamins and Supplements

Gastric bypass surgery allows food to bypass the part of the small intestine where many nutrients, minerals, and vitamins are most easily absorbed. Therefore, taking vitamins and supplements after surgery is advised. According to the American Society for Metabolic and Bariatric Surgery (ASMBS), anemia and osteoporosis are the most common long-term complications of the RNY gastric bypass surgery because both calcium and iron absorption is reduced when the intestines are bypassed. Therefore, it is essential for patients to be closely monitored and lifetime supplementation is necessary. Other deficiencies may occur such as Vitamin B 1 (thiamine), Vitamin B 12, and Vitamin D.

It is essential to consume a protein and nutrient-rich diet in addition to taking vitamins. To avoid deficiencies it may be necessary to take specially formulated or additional vitamins (A, D, E, and K in water-soluble form).

It is thought that as much as 50 percent of people in the United States have a vitamin D deficiency, but gastric bypass patients are at a higher risk. Bone disease such as osteoporosis can occur because of the reduced capacity to absorb calcium. However, the risk of osteoporosis can be decreased with calcium and vitamin D supplements.

Vitamin E deficiency, although rare, can occur with fat mal-absorption. Symptoms include poor nerve function that causes numbness or tingling, muscle weakness, poor vision, and decreased ability to fight infections.

Hypocalcemia

Hypocalcemia is a medical term for low levels of calcium due to vitamin D deficiency. Calcium and iron deficiencies are possible due to the body's limited absorption ability after mal-absorption surgeries. These deficiencies can cause bone loss and fractures.

Calcium citrate is mandatory, not only due to an altered anatomy, but also based on the fact that there is less hydrochloric acid present in a smaller stomach. Calcium citrate is better absorbed in this environment.

Iron is best absorbed in the elemental form. It is recommended that calcium and iron be taken at least 2 hours apart since they compete for absorption. Menstrual cycles can increase the risk for anemia and pre-menopausal women could be advised to take higher dosages (prenatal amounts) of iron since ongoing blood loss is a factor.

After mal-absorption surgery, it is strongly recommended that patients take daily vitamin and mineral supplements to prevent nutritional complications.

It is important to note that taking any vitamins, minerals, or supplements should be based on an individual blood test and should be taken under the advice of your physician.

I find it easier to take vitamins and other supplements when I put them in a pill organizer case. It is convenient to fill several cases at one time. Because several medications and supplements must be taken several hours apart, I send reminders to myself on my phone. This can be done on your calendar or with a phone application.

Protein Priority

Mal-absorptive surgeries will require that you add a higher gram count of quality protein to your diet. This is recommended for the long-term. In the beginning, this elevation in dietary protein will change forms from primary liquid supplements, to adding more real, whole food proteins into your diet (from the weight loss phase and into maintenance).

Steatorrhea

Some side effects of surgery can be avoided; but there are a few side effects that are caused by mal-absorption that cannot be avoided. Because our systems don't digest foods as well as they used to, when undigested food and undigested fats reaches our colon, the enzymes and bacteria go a little wild and crazy trying to digest it. Known as steatorrhea—this mal-absorption issue causes frequent bowel movements, unpredictable diarrhea, and excessive and foul smelling gas. Most post-surgery patients are desperate to find a solution to this embarrassment. Having dealt with embarrassment for most of our lives, the unfortunate reality is there is not much we can do to eliminate this side effect. However, it may help to eliminate or limit certain foods from your diet that are more prone to forming gas.

Frequent loose stools can potentially increase the risk of dehydration. Constipation may also result after surgery. Both loose stools and constipation are quite normal after surgery and are usually temporary.

Additional Medical Abdominal and Intestinal Issues

Learning how to care for and protect your newly-formed pouch from ulcers and other medical complications is not to be taken lightly. These can produce life-threatening complications.

Ulcers

Ulcers are a much more serious complication after gastric bypass surgery because the new pouch will be very tiny. There is literally no room for ulcers. Getting off of caffeine, alcohol, and nicotine is required (hopefully you did this before surgery.) These create an acidic environment for the body, which can compromise your stomach pouch by putting you at risk for developing ulcers. Nicotine also slows the healing process.

Some medications also put you at risk for ulcers. (see Medication Do's and Don'ts.)

Bowel Obstruction

Rerouting the bowel carries risk for bowel obstruction. Abdominal pain could be a symptom of a bowel obstruction. Any abdominal pain should never be overlooked. Notify your surgeon or get medical attention immediately if you experience any pain in this area.

Medication Do's and Don'ts

It is paramount to learn about medications you can and can't take after gastric bypass procedures and how they will affect your new pouch.

There are certain medications that gastric bypass patients

should NOT take, including NSAIDS and steroids. NSAIDS are non-steroidal anti-inflammatory drugs and include ibuprofen, (e.g. Advil, Motrin, and Aleve). Medications, such as steroids are commonly given for pain and inflammation. Gastric bypass patients shouldn't take these medications because they are at a higher risk for ulcers, and NSAIDS significantly increase the risk of ulcers. Oral steroids should not be taken without medical supervision and prescription medications to protect the pouch. Your surgeon should provide you with a list of other significant medications that must be avoided. *(There is a list provided on the Miles to Go Blog at www.milestogoblog.com.)*

A New Medical MO

Modus Operandi, or MO, for short. That's Latin for "method of operating," meaning the normal operating procedures. But as weight loss surgery recipients, our parts don't operate by the normal method anymore and neither does our medical care. After surgery, some medical methods of operation change for us as well as information we should share with emergency, hospital, or other health care professionals.

From now on, any time you receive medical care, *ANY and ALL* medical personnel who are treating you need to know that you have had weight loss surgery and what kind of procedure you had. It is always of the utmost importance. It could save your life.

When it comes to emergencies, time is of the essence. Knowing your history, an informed medical staff will help ensure that you get proper medical treatment without unnecessary delays. Knowing that you are a weight loss surgery patient lets them know certain medical conditions to look for that they might not check on a non-weight loss surgery patient. Depending on your symptoms, they could look for things such as vitamin and mineral deficiencies, ulcers, bowel obstruction, and imbalanced blood sugar levels.

Medical protocol will differ from other patients. After weight loss surgery, there are certain medical procedures that should be altered, such as using smaller-diameter instruments. You may want to consider wearing medical identification.

No Ifs, Ands, or Butts About It

Lifestyle change includes quitting smoking. I don't have to tell you how many harmful ingredients cigarettes contain or how many harmful effects smoking has on the body. You probably already realize that.

I will say that although there are more than 4,000 hazardous compounds present in cigarette smoke, there are additional health concerns in smoking other than just addiction, poison, pollution, and disease. Smoking affects the body's ability to heal and stay healthy after weight loss surgery.

Smoking decreases the amount of oxygen, while increasing the amount of carbon monoxide in your blood. Carbon monoxide makes your heart pump less efficiently, and limits your body's overall oxygen supply. The nicotine consumed increases your need for oxygen. So, while oxygen supply is being limited, your body demands more oxygen. Without enough oxygen, it is much harder to heal.

This can lead to serious healing complications, including excessive bleeding, infection, tissue death, increased risk of cardiovascular complications, and heart weakness. Smoking also increases inflammation, clogs the lungs, shrinks your body's airways, and makes your lungs more prone to collapse.

According to a study at the Johns Hopkins School of Medicine, nicotine also affects the brain and your ability to sleep. The study showed that smokers experienced less deep sleep. This stage of sleep in which the body repairs itself and heals wounds. Deep sleep also affects the body's muscle mass, metabolism, and overall health.

The Balance Of Life

Exercise is always an amusing consideration for an overweight person. Just getting up out of a chair takes planning and strategy that most folks never consider. Ah, but activity and exercise involve more than that, although getting up out of the chair is the first step. Exercise to the overweight is not only humiliating, but they seem to mix like oil and water.

Committing to an exercise routine as well as increased physical activity is an extremely important element for reaching your weight loss goal. I have found that exercise and activity are necessary to the weight loss phase and crucial for maintaining weight loss long-term. But exercise strengthens more than our body; it also strengthens our mind and our spirit.

I once read a book by Richard Exley, *"The Rhythm of Life."* I was impressed by his "balanced" approach to life as an integrated whole. I began to understand the importance of making balance a priority and adopted this perspective into my own life. Exley shares how much more fulfilled our lives would be if we included a more equally incorporated experience of work, rest, worship, and play into our lives. Created in the likeness of God, the biblical commandments institute these principles for us. Exley states, *"I believe work can be meaningful, rest can renew, worship can inspire, and play can be the joyous pleasure that seasons it all."*

Even our play can offer rewarding benefits such as physical exercise, relief stress, as well as enhance relationships. Whether a class at the gym, training for a marathon, a leisure stroll, a recreational game of volleyball, a day of sailing, canoeing, fishing with friends, or a round of golf with a loved one; activity, exercise, and play can be gratifying as well as profitable.

Studies show that exercise reduces anxiety resulting in more sound sleep. Both sleep and exercise allow us to think more clearly and handle life's challenges more successfully.

In the pre-surgery phase, we reviewed the elements of setting goals, forming a plan of action, and finding the necessary

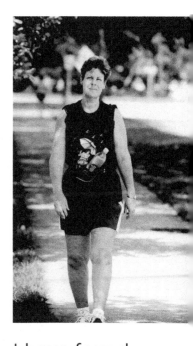

I have found that exercise and activity are necessary to the weight loss phase and crucial for maintaining weight loss long-term.

motivation that will keep us active and healthy. I used to play a lot of golf, but over the years my activities, goals, and exercises have changed. Aside from overall health benefits of exercise, my most recent goals are to stay strong and flexible as I age. I have had to find types of exercises in which I am willing to make a commitment. Several days a week, I go to the gym and use the equipment, do some weight lifting, and occasionally join in an exercise class. I might add in some bike riding and walking, when my schedule and the weather permits. I do these because I am motivated to stay healthy. But I have found one that I enjoy more than any other—Pilates. Pilates is defined as a series of non-impact exercises to develop strength, flexibility, and balance. Aside from helping me meet my goal, I look forward to attending classes each week.

I urge you to start simple and find enjoyable activities that motivate you and keep you going strong for the rest of your life.

Follow-up with Long-term Medical Care

Sometimes we tend to think that we are on this road alone, but we are not, we have the opportunity to follow others as they lead us into success.

Following in someone's footsteps, suggests that someone has been down the path before us, giving us a more reliable path. It means that we accept their beliefs and trust them to lead us safely to our destination. Following involves pursuing with loyalty and commitment, as they encourage us to reach deep and find the stamina to keep going even if the road does get bumpy. It gives us the opportunity to learn from those who have overcome adversity, thus giving us inspiration and strength.

In order to follow, we must hold our head up, turn our eyes upward and forget what is behind, focus on what is just ahead.

This includes the team of professionals whom you selected for your pre-surgery care and life-altering surgery. They, no doubt, are leaders in the fields of bariatrics, nutrition, and healthcare who are trained to excel in their profession. If you *followed* their advice with your pre-surgery care needs, why not *follow* afterwards with post-surgery care?

New medical discoveries are continually being made, and this is why your multidisciplinary team is extremely important in this process. Committing to lifelong follow-up with a bariatric medical care professional for medical updates, including yearly blood work is crucial for our long-term health.

Follow-up visits decrease post-operative complications and maximize weight loss. A study of 208 gastric bypass and 201 gastric banding patients revealed that patients who followed guidelines after surgery lost 35 percent more weight in the year following surgery than those who didn't. The study also showed that patients who received follow-up care remained compliant and kept more weight off for the long term.

I strongly encourage you to commit to long-term care after surgery. Your team of bariatric professionals is committed to your long-term post-operative care and it is just as important as your pre-surgery care—if not more important.

Follow the leaders of your professional support team as they lead you onward to a lifetime of permanent success. Overtake those thoughts of complacency. Reach forward to capture your dreams and make them a reality. Continue your pursuit of health by *following* bariatric guidelines and *follow up* with yearly checkups.

You can lead the way for others to follow. So don't give up, be persistent and courageous and follow the advice of your health-care professionals.

Committing to lifelong follow-up with a bariatric medical care professional for medical updates, including yearly blood work is crucial for our long-term health.

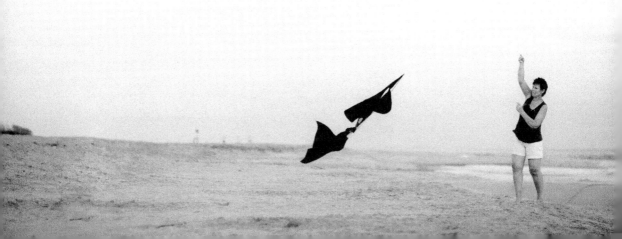

Out of Obesity by Julia Holloman

CHAPTER 26

V. Honor Thy New (Altered) Reality

**Things turn out best for the people who
make the best out of the way things turn out.**

Art Linkletter

Now that we understand the physical changes that take place
after weight loss surgery and the importance of taking care of our
new body, there are other issues we need to examine.

Along with weight loss came changes in my body from head
to toe. Although most health related illnesses are improved or
even dissipate after losing weight, there are some that *aren't
resolved*. There are even issues that are actually *created* by
surgery and losing weight. Experiencing these conditions can
bring feelings of disappointment and frustration, especially if
we are expecting unrealistic or idealistic results. Success after
weight loss also includes accepting your altered anatomy and
the resulting "new you."

It is tempting to think that after you lose weight, life will be
perfect. However, neither life, nor our body, will be as perfect as we
imagine. Although we can find success with weight loss surgery, it
is neither a time machine nor a miracle worker.

Remember how the Israelites idealized their former life in
Egypt? We are most likely dreaming of returning to the life we
had before obesity or maybe even an idealized version of what
we think life will be like. *"If only I could get back to the body I had*

when I was 18, 21, ____" (you fill in the blank). We cannot expect our body to return to a perfect, flawless ideal. No one has a perfect body—not before, or after.

Our body has been changing throughout our entire life. We can't expect to go back to what was before. Unless we want to return to obesity, and our unhealthy lifestyle, we must go forward.

Sooner or later, we must face the truth. This is where another aspect of acceptance must be allowed to take place. We must let go of what used to be, depart from an unrealistic expectation of weight loss, and abandon the unrealistic desire to return to our distorted version of perfection. We took a risk and paid a price for improved health. These are the consequences we accepted when we chose to have an elective life-altering surgery. This is our new body and our new reality.

During these times, it has been especially helpful for me to remember what my quality of life was like before and appreciate the overall benefits of losing weight and gaining health. Yes, things in the new place will be different. I left the former behind. Surgery offered me a chance to start over in a brand new place. The new place holds riches and great rewards beyond measure. However, I have had to learn to accept the "although improved, not so perfect, leftover me!"

> ...it has been especially helpful for me to remember what my quality of life was like before and appreciate the overall benefits of losing weight and gaining health.

Goodbye Waves

One of the challenges after surgery is dealing with the fear of hair loss. Regardless of whether you are male or female, losing your hair is an emotional experience in and of itself. Although, we lose hair everyday, we may experience a little more than our normal hair loss during the weight loss phase.

Although the exact reason for hair loss is unknown, massive weight loss tends to disrupt our hair's natural growth process. In addition, hormonal changes, medication, as well as stress from healing, changes in diet, and anesthesia from surgery may also play a part. So don't add additional stress to your life by worrying about hair loss.

The amount of hair loss varies from individual to individual. About 20 to 30 percent of patients experience hair loss of some sort after banding and a majority after gastric bypass. Hair loss usually occurs between three to six months after surgery, during the time when the greatest weight loss is experienced. Even if you are following the guidelines of good nutrition, it is probable that you will experience hair loss.

Now, let's hear the good news.

Although hair loss may be concerning, you can rest assured it is temporary. Returning to better health increases the possibility for healthier hair.

I haven't missed too many support group meetings since my first visit, in February of 2006, and I remember being impressed by how healthy those who had undergone surgery looked. For the most part, I couldn't believe those who had reached their goal weight were *EVER* overweight. They had healthy skin, and I didn't recognize any thinning hair or hair loss.

Most of the time when we are going through the hair loss stage of weight loss, we think it is evident to everyone. The fact is, *most of the time* it's not obvious to others. It may *"appear"* that all of our hair is falling out, but it's not, and chances are very high that we won't go bald. Honestly, no one will know but you.

In view of the larger picture of returning to a greater health and renewed life, hair loss is relatively insignificant.

There are ways we can take care of our hair during this weight loss phase as well as promote healthier hair for the long-term. Jina Banner, a cosmetologist at Della Testa Hair Salon, here in Wilmington, NC, says, *"Our hair is our best accessory, and we wear it everyday."* Jina offers these suggestions to ease the worries of hair loss.

- Healthy hair is a sign of good overall health. Eat a well-balanced diet. (Getting 60 to 100 grams of protein each day is recommended by medical professionals.)
- Take the recommended vitamins and minerals suggested

by your surgeon to avoid deficiencies. These may include zinc, iron, calcium, Vitamin E, A, and Biotin (which is a B vitamin). Vitamin B helps your body deal with stress along with a balance of exercise, sleep, and relaxation.

- If you have stopped smoking, you have also lowered your risk of hair loss.
- Wet hair is more fragile, combing and brushing wet hair weakens it. When drying wet hair, Jina says our fingers are our best tools. Lifting gently, dry wet hair using your fingers until slightly damp. Finish styling with a brush or comb.
- Getting regular haircuts promotes growth and keeps hair healthy. As you lose weight the shape of your face changes. You might consider getting a new updated hairstyle that is best fitted to your new emerging personality and your new face shape, especially during the weight loss phase.
- Hair products can also increase the health of your hair. Jina suggests Nioxen—a line of hair care products that include vitamins, conditioners, shampoos, and scalp sprays.

Returning to better health increases the possibly for healthier hair. So, be encouraged and remember, even though hair loss is probable, it is also temporary. As weight loss slows down, hair loss slows down.

Let's Get Personal

Experts say there may be more than 60 hormones in the human body. As we grow older, our hormones fluctuate. Just like weight affects our outward physical body, our weight can also cause fluctuations in our reproductive hormones. These hormone imbalances affect us physically, as well as emotionally, mentally, psychologically, and sexually.

Changes in these hormones can be beneficial and annoying. It's important to understand the transitions that are taking place as we experience massive weight loss.

For women, estrogen is stored in our fat cells. The more fat cells there are in the body, the more estrogen is produced and the more we store. (Excess weight that is stored in the belly is an indicator of high levels of estrogen.) Unfortunately, high levels of estrogen in fat cells can also hinder the body's ability to burn fat, which makes it more difficult to lose weight.

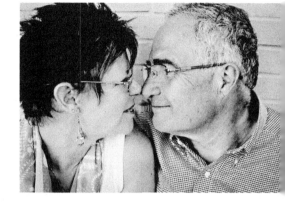

When we lose weight, we lose fat cells. When we lose fat cells, we lose estrogen stores. Lowering estrogen levels triggers changes in the body. These symptoms are frequently associated with menopause and can vary widely. Sometimes these symptoms can be quite subtle and sometimes they can be downright horrendous. Symptoms include fatigue, hot flashes, night sweats, memory lapses, difficulty concentrating, joint pain, vaginal dryness, dry skin, and loss of libido, just to name a few.

Having had a hysterectomy previously, I had to discontinue my hormone replacement therapy, in preparation for gastric bypass. After surgery, I made the decision not to go back on the hormones. But several months later, I began to experience some of these hormonal related difficulties. I thought I was going crazy and felt like my body was falling apart. Let's just say, there is nothing sexy about imbalanced hormones and sexual dysfunction. Did I lose weight for this? I don't think so. After doing some research and consulting with a gynecologist, I returned to the hormone replacement therapy. My symptoms dissipated and life returned to normal. Actually, life got better than my before surgery normal.

Hormonal changes are not all bad. According to research presented by the American Society for Metabolic & Bariatric Surgery, close to 70 percent of women who have weight loss surgery see improvements in their sex lives within six months. Hormonal changes not only affect women, but men as well. Both men and women report better sexual function after losing weight.

Shanu N. Kothari, MD, a bariatric surgeon at Gundersen Lutheran in La Crosse, Wisconsin says that we focus on so many obesity-related comorbid conditions such as high blood pressure, diabetes, and sleep apnea, that we tend to overlook other quality of life issues that are affected by weight loss—such as sexual dysfunction. He says that sexual dysfunction is one of the "hidden" comorbid conditions that can improve with weight loss surgery.

Researcher Dale Bond, PhD, assistant professor of psychiatry and human behavior at Miriam Hospital Weight Control and Diabetes Research Center at Brown University Medical School says, *"Exactly why the women's sex lives improved after weight loss surgery is not fully understood, but several factors, including improved body image and mood, as well as changes in their hormonal profile, may play a role."*

John W. Baker, MD, president of the American Society for Metabolic & Bariatric Surgery and the medical director of the Baptist Medical Center's Health Weight Loss Center in Little Rock, Arkansas, says that sexual function may be just the tip of the iceberg. *"We also see improvements in infertility and reductions in complications related to pregnancy in women who have bariatric surgery."* He also states that men, too, reap similar benefits. *"Males tend to have improved testosterone (male sex hormone) levels and related improvements in energy, drive, and function."*

It's important to listen to your body and learn all you can about the changes you are going through. Do your homework, educate yourself on changes in your body, be willing to find solutions, and team up with your health-care professionals to return to optimal health.

The Left-Over Me: Changes from Head to Toe

As we lose weight, our body goes through many physical changes that are often unanticipated. With the increase of bariatric surgery comes the increase in changes that can be experienced by patients after surgery. These changes not only baffle bariatric patients, I also found they can puzzle the most qualified professionals.

I had eye surgery to correct my far vision before having bariatric surgery. I knew I would have to wear reading glasses, but I was so disappointed when I realized that my intermediate vision was changing and my eye exams revealed I needed to start wearing glasses again. This wasn't just a slight change; but for a few months my near vision was changing so rapidly that by the time my new glasses had come in and I got adjusted to them, I would have to go back for a re-check and start all over again. This went on for several months.

I discovered that although my overall health affected my eyes, massive weight loss also played a significant role in my vision. My eye care professional, Dr. Tracey Glendenning, says, "*Studies have shown that eye complications can occur from sudden weight loss and dietary changes. Now there's evidence that gastric bypass surgery may be connected. With these changes, patients may experience a vitamin deficiency, which can cause poor night vision, corneal, and cataract changes. A lack of vitamin C and E may cause premature cataracts. Patients should maintain adequate vitamin supplementation post gastric bypass.*"

My dental work also changed. The bridge in my mouth started to feel different. The gum under my bridge had gotten smaller, so there was more space between my gum and my tooth. It felt like I was missing a tooth. It took a while before it felt normal again. My dentist was amazed, they don't usually see this happen, but how often does someone lose 164 pounds?

My friend Robin told me that her gums and dental work had also changed, as well as her eyes. She has lost over 380 pounds and has done a fabulous job of maintaining that for over 6 years. You go, girl!

I remember the feeling when I suddenly realized that there was actually space between my legs when I walked. That felt very strange.

My shoe size changed. Before, I was wearing a 9 1/2 and thinking that 10's would be more comfortable. But as my grandmother always said, "*Pride never gets too hot or too cold.*" I guess my pride wouldn't let me look for larger ones! I had resigned just to wear uncomfortable shoes or go without. Good thing we live in a warmer climate where sandals and flip-flops can go almost year-round. Now, I usually wear an 8 and sometimes a 7 ½ or even a 7, which is the size I wore when I got married at age 18. How strange and unexpectedly wonderful.

Changes are just a part of the process. Some have been thrilling and just down right amazing, while others seem terribly inconvenient and annoying.

Baby, It's Cold Outside

If there is one thing about weight loss that sends shivers down my spine, it's just that. I'm cold. All the time. So, I did a little research to find out why, and what do you know, there really is a scientific reason.

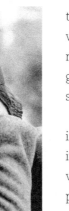

Our body has two ways of regulating temperature: sweating and shivering. Before weight loss, I knew a lot about sweating or, maybe I should use a more ladylike term, glistening! Nevertheless, we exchange that for a slimmer body, less insulation and—the shivers.

While losing weight, our body is losing its insulation and also generating less energy because it doesn't have to work as hard to carry the extra weight. It seems that our body's metabolic cell processes have also slowed down.

Scientifically speaking, as our extremities cool, our body re-routes blood flow to our core, in its response to keeping our vital organs at an optimal temperature. As the temperature falls, our feet, legs, arms, and hands may get cooler.

Most weight loss patients report that their body temperature stabilizes in about 24 months; but I'm well past that, and I'm still shivering. It was also reported that people who exercised regularly were warmer and shivered less. Nice try, but I didn't warm up with that idea, either.

I'm so glad the layered look is in, because I'm wearing lots of new layers. These layers are easier to remove than weight and are nice and warm. So, bring on winter (or anything cooler than 75 degrees for that matter, including air conditioning) because I've always got an extra sweater in my purse and my car. Along with those stylish scarves, gloves, camis, sweaters, and multiple layers of clothing, including my new favorite—leg warmers.

It may be a little chilly on the outside, but as I've taken off that extra layer of interior insulation, I can now add on stylish new layers of clothing instead.

A Problem with My Coccyx

My what? My coccyx. You know, your tailbone, the one at the end of your spinal column. The one you sit on.

I thought surely I had a growth or some severe malady on my spine. I made appointments with several doctors. But after many conversations and a set of x-rays, they each assured me I had no abnormal growth or problems.

I was sent home to sit on a doughnut for a few months. Well, I guess if I can't eat them I might as well sit on them. No, I mean a pillow with a hole in it. After months of carrying that embarrassing pillow around wherever I went, I was still in severe pain.

Then one day, while walking with a weight loss surgery friend, I mentioned the issue. As it turned out, she had the same problem herself and discovered that after surgery she had to improve her balance and muscular strength in her legs and learn to walk differently. She suggested I see a physical therapist.

I discovered that being overweight as well as changes in weight and hormones had affected my muscles and my sitting posture. Having weak muscles around the tailbone or coccyx causes too much movement, which in turn affected my tailbone, and it had

215

become irritated. Part of my basic therapy was doing Pilates to strengthen the muscles around the tailbone and it helped heal the irritation and my coccyx. Afterwards, I could even sit with my legs up and balance on my tailbone. Maybe that's more than you wanted to know, but here is something you might want to know.

Poor balance combined with loss of muscular strength in the legs are why falls in the elderly are so common. Pilates strengthens your body's core muscles around the spine.

Moral of the story: having a problem with your coccyx is a pain in the...tailbone. Throw out **all** the doughnuts, find a good physical therapist, and enroll in Pilates Classes.

It's Time to Wake Up

Following weight loss surgery, there are lots of things we have had to give up. However, there are some things that we may have given up that we shouldn't have—and one of them is our CPAP.

Before surgery, many of us are extremely concerned about the fatalities related to having weight loss surgery, and rightly so. But, few are as concerned about giving up their CPAP machine, which is also life-threatening. We need to wake up to the dangers of sleep apnea.

My passion for helping others find success after weight loss surgery includes continued awareness associated with sleep apnea. If you have been diagnosed with sleep apnea and have been given a prescription for a Continuous Positive Airway Pressure machine (CPAP), to treat this condition, there are several facts you should know.

- Sleep apnea may not be resolved by losing weight.
- Sleep apnea can be fatal.
- Sleep apnea can cause obesity.
- Obesity can cause sleep apnea.
- There are different types of sleep apnea.
- Not all of types of sleep apnea are caused by being overweight.

Types of Sleep Apnea

Sleep Apnea is a sleep disorder characterized by abnormal pauses in breathing or instances of abnormally low breathing during sleep. Each pause in breathing, called an *apnea*, can last from a few seconds to minutes, and may occur 5 to 30 times or more an hour. Similarly, each abnormally low breathing event is called a *hypopnea*. *Hypoxia* is a deficiency in the amount of oxygen reaching body tissues.

There are three types of sleep apnea. The most common type is *obstructive sleep apnea* (OSA). The less common type is *central sleep apnea* (CSA). The third less common type is *mixed sleep apnea*, which is basically a combination of OSA and CSA.

OSA, is caused by the relaxation and collapsing of the soft tissue at the back of the throat which blocks the passage of air into the lungs and results in the frequent stoppage of breathing during sleep. Snoring is caused by vibrations of the relaxed throat tissues and is often the precursor to or companion of sleep apnea.

CSA is a brain-related condition. CSA occurs without snoring and is not caused by an obstruction. Rather, it is caused by the failure of the brain to signal for a breath.

Although weight can aggravate this condition, these types of muscle-related and brain-related sleep apneas are not cured by weight loss.

As you can see, sleep apnea is not always caused by weight. Therefore, **losing weight is not considered a cure for sleep apnea.** Weight loss sometimes *lessens* the obstruction in your throat and on your diaphragm; so your episodes could improve, but seldom is this condition resolved completely. Unless you were diagnosed with a very mild case of OSA, chances are very low that losing weight will resolve it.

Don't assume that because you have lost weight or that the air pressure of your CPAP machine has become too strong that you don't need it. It is also very dangerous to assume you have been cured. Many people have sleep apnea and don't know it. Sleep apnea may occur over a long period of time before people become

> ...sleep apnea is not always caused by weight. Therefore, **losing weight is not considered a cure for sleep apnea.**

aware of it and seek medical treatment. The only way to tell is to get re-tested.

If you were diagnosed with sleep apnea and are not wearing your CPAP machine for any reason, except for a re-test that medically proves you are cured (before or after weight loss), it's time to wake up. Prematurely giving up your CPAP increases the chance that you might not *wake up* at all.

I Didn't Know

I was diagnosed with sleep apnea in 2004, about two years before weight loss surgery. I did not know I had it. Actually, I ignored the signs. I was in denial. That was until several years later when I couldn't make up the bed without feeling like I had run a marathon.

It was only after getting a CPAP machine that I realized how badly I really did feel. I had blamed a lot of my symptoms on just being overweight. Chances are I had it before I became severely overweight. Maybe it even added to the problem.

It is reported that 95 percent of the millions of people who suffer from sleep apnea have not and may never be diagnosed, let alone treated.

Don't Give Up

Like most of us, I fully expected to give up my CPAP after weight loss, but, as it turned out, I still needed it.

According to a study published in the *Journal of Clinical Sleep Medicine*, 24 severely-obese adults were tested for obstructive sleep apnea before and after getting weight loss surgery and again a year later. Even though the patients trimmed their BMI from 51 to 32, a year later they were still obese—even though a lot less than before bariatric surgery. The study found that only one of the patients no longer had obstructive sleep apnea a year after surgery.

Their sleep apnea was changed after surgery, their symptoms eased to varying degrees, but not enough to end their obstructive sleep apnea. All of the other patients with obstructive sleep apnea still needed a CPAP machine to help them breathe better at night. Only six of these patients were using their CPAP machines.

Based on a seven and a half year study by the *American College of Chest Physicians* on sleep apnea and morbidly-obese patients following weight loss surgery, the conclusion is this: "*We conclude that morbid obesity is not the only causative factor in the sleep apnea syndrome for these patients. Weight reduction surgery alone does not "cure" their sleep apnea, and they are still at risk.*"

After losing weight, I could not handle the air pressure of my machine and I thought I was cured. I eliminated my CPAP on my own and I was sleeping pretty well, or so I thought. After a period of time, I began experiencing extreme fatigue and morning headaches, and discovered that my sleep apnea had not been resolved.

My sleep apnea episodes are fewer and are not as severe as I had before losing weight, but I still have it.

I didn't realize how many times my sleep was being disturbed until after returning to the CPAP machine. I lost weight and gained more energy.

Risk of Sleep Apnea

We need sleep for many important reasons, including weight loss and brain function. I don't know about you, but I need all the help I can get in these two areas.

Rest, sleep, and relaxation are just as important for bringing life into proper balance as activity, recreation, and proper diet.

Sleep comes in several stages, one of which is REM sleep. It is the period when we dream. During REM sleep, our mind is on hyper-alert and our body experiences low muscle tone. (This keeps us from jumping out of bed during our dreams).

REM is important because this is when our thoughts are organized and creativity is nourished. While you sleep, your brain is reviewing all the things that you have done or learned during the day. It is reviewing, sorting, organizing, prioritizing, problem-solving, and memorizing. When it comes to being smarter, you only lose if you don't snooze.

Sleep also controls our metabolism. A lack of sleep is associated with imbalanced levels of the hormones that are involved in the regulation of body fat, hunger control, and satiety. During sleep the body also replaces appetite-related hormones.

Sleep apnea deprives us of REM sleep. So, if you wear your CPAP you do lose—weight that is! To lose or not to lose, that is the question!

Sleep deprivation affects your energy level, ability to concentrate, and may result in many transportation accidents and fatalities.

Sleep apnea can put you at risk for liver disease, heart disease, heart attacks, diabetes, high blood pressure, and other health risks. It can also result in low metabolism and ineffective weight loss. Its risks are considered to rank with smoking, obesity, high cholesterol, and high blood pressure.

Many of the dangers of sleep apnea are related to how your heart functions. In a study of about 11,000 adults, researchers found that sleep apnea was the second biggest risk for sudden death among heart disease patients.

Pauses in breathing during sleep that characterize sleep apnea can cause drastic changes in your oxygen levels and blood pressure. When this happens, it puts a strain on the heart as it shuts off oxygen to the brain and body and increases your risk of stroke. Research shows that people with sleep apnea are more likely to have high blood pressure, and are two to four times more likely to have a stroke.

Research has now found that repeated surges and drops in blood pressure and low oxygen levels eventually impair the body's ability to regulate blood flow to the brain.

Studies also show that CPAP may reduce blood pressure levels in people with sleep apnea. The continuous use of CPAP over an extended period of time may also help protect, as well as reduce, the risks of such heart problems as congestive heart failure, coronary artery disease, irregular heartbeat, and stroke.

We need more sleep than we think. A national experiment revealed that in the 1850's, the average person got nine and a half hours of sleep per night. By 1910, the average per night was seven hours. Today, we get two and a half hours less sleep than 150 years ago. One-third of us get less than six hours of sleep per night. In a poll done by the *American Medical News* in 1999, 27 percent of the general population admitted to falling asleep while driving just within that year.

What You Can Do

Those who make up their mind to wear the CPAP apparatus have less trouble and are able to adjust more quickly. Partial use keeps the body from getting fully adjusted to the machine and also puts your health at risk. I can tell you from experience that the more I wear the CPAP mask, the more I can tolerate it. Here are some suggestions that might help make it easier to tolerate your CPAP machine.

- Find a mask that works for you. It's the mask that is the key to success. Update your mask often. Oils from your skin can cause the seal of the mask to break down over several months of use. Check with your insurance company regarding coverage costs of updated equipment and supplies. Keep trying until you find the mask that you can tolerate and fits properly by experimenting with different sizes and styles.
- You might find it helpful to make a change in your sleep position or find a pillow that works better with your mask.
- Get your pressure checked often to make sure it is at the right level for you. If your CPAP pressure needs adjusting, a medical doctor can give you a prescription that will allow a respiratory therapist to make adjustments in your airway pressure.

- Update your machine. The CPAP machine has changed so much in the last few years. My doctor prescribed an auto-titration machine. This machine senses upcoming episodes and automatically adjusts the pressure accordingly.

There are humidifiers, chin straps, filters, alarm clocks, and even music available on these machines now. So, go try out the latest versions and get all the bells and whistles.

On occasion, I take my machine to the therapist who checks the information card on the machine to see if the mask is fitting properly, if there are any leaks, how many episodes I have, how much pressure the machine is supplying, and if any adjustments need to be made. Amazing! No more guessing.

The unfortunate reality is that after weight loss surgery, you may have sleep apnea or other health issues that are not resolved by losing weight. It will be important to learn to take care of your new body and your new self.

Armed with information and a renewed focus on life, you can breathe easier, while returning to renewed health and vitality.

Late Dumping Syndrome

Gastric bypass surgery does carry risk; but late dumping was one I was unaware of in the beginning. Professionals are still making new discoveries about what happens to our body when it is altered.

Just when you thought that early dumping syndrome was over and you find that you can tolerate more sugar, there may be another form of dumping that can occur.

Dumping syndrome comes in two stages, both early and late. Depending on the occurrence of symptoms in relation to the time elapsed after a meal. Both forms occur when a rapid delivery of large amounts of undigested foods enter the intestines. Symptoms may vary widely from patient to patient.

Although as the names imply, early dumping occurs early in the weight loss process for gastric bypass patients, and late dumping occurs several years later.

Late dumping syndrome is a result of low blood sugar caused by excess insulin produced in response to sudden dumping of food and fluids, such as sugar or carbohydrates, into the intestine. Late dumping occurs two hours after eating and can occur much later in the process, one to three years after weight loss surgery.

It will be a very good idea to limit your sugar intake. My experience is that late dumping can sneak up on you without warning—and being "*late*" is never timely!

Symptoms of late dumping syndrome include profuse sweating, anxiety, and tremors. Headache, exhaustion, and fainting may occur. It can also include an urgency to eat. This is not the same urgency that is associated with emotional hunger; this is caused by your body's physical need for fuel.

This low drop in blood sugar is also known as hypoglycemia. Hypoglycemia after weight loss surgery is common, and is usually mild and can be corrected with dietary changes. Severe cases of reactive hypoglycemia after gastric bypass surgery are rare. It only takes a small change to get things off balance when you have an altered digestive system and, for some of us, that threshold may be more sensitive than for others.

If you think you may have symptoms of low blood sugar it is important to seek medical attention. Hypoglycemia is a potentially dangerous condition, so it is very important to know the signs and effects of low blood sugar. If your dumping episodes are not controlled by diet and become severe, you will need to inform a health-care professional.

Although carbohydrate sensitivity is common after surgery and can most often be controlled by diet, severe hypoglycemia is rare. In one percent of those who suffer from severe hypoglycemia, it cannot be controlled by diet alone. In these cases, prescribed medications, adjustments in daily activity, alongside carefully monitoring of one's diet, can help to stabilize drops in blood sugar.

The Ups and Downs of Plateaus

In the beginning, the surgery will do most of the work and weight loss expectations are high. But let's face it. Not only do we want things to be easy, but we also want weight loss to happen *fast*. We have grown accustomed to expecting things in our lives to happen right away. We live in a culture of fast food, instant coffee, text messaging, and drive thru windows at every stop. So, just like every diet we have ever been on, the expectation is that the result will be massive weight loss in a hurry, and this is especially so after bariatric surgery.

Compliance assures us that weight loss WILL happen. But there is no guarantee that weight loss will be fast or continuous— even with the assist of surgery. This process must include an "expectation adjustment."

During the weight loss phase, we should expect a wide range of experiences alongside massive weight loss.

During the weight loss phase, we should expect a wide range of experiences alongside massive weight loss. Weight loss surgery patient, Barbara Thompson, has written several books about weight loss surgery. She points out that, *"True weight loss consists of three phases: weight loss, plateaus and small weight regains."* It is just a normal part of the process.

A plateau is defined as a place that is level and stable. Well, our weight may be stable, but experiencing a weight loss plateau, especially after bariatric surgery, is anything but stable emotionally. Plateaus can send us on an emotional roller coaster. And, just like the real roller coaster, they can be quite alarming. If you're like me, the only plateau I like is the one that comes after I have lost all the weight I want to lose, not before. But plateaus don't just show up, they often arrive sooner than we expect and stay longer than we wish.

This is an individual journey, and our body responds differently both surgically and nutritionally. Everyone will lose at a different pace. Even so, it will be important to understand the weight loss process, know what we can expect, and be equipped to emerge victorious.

Understanding the Process

In the beginning, weight loss may be fast. Remember, at first we are in the *"honeymoon phase"* of weight loss. During this period of time the weight seems to come off almost without effort. This *"honeymoon phase"* and is our *"window of opportunity"* to lose the most weight. But even here in this phase, we can encounter a few plateaus. Early on, plateaus are usually short-lived and weight loss continues.

For gastric bypass patients, this *"weight loss window"* begins to close around the end of the first year to eighteen months, and weight loss will gradually begin to slow.

Weight plateaus typically occur around 18 to 24 months, but at any time throughout the process it is not out of the ordinary to experience a plateau. It is totally normal for weight loss to slow, come to a standstill, or even go up from time to time. These fluctuations occur as the body adjusts and recalculates its position.

Even as weight loss slows, with diligent compliance to diet and exercise, we can continue to lose weight and move toward our goal weight.

My bariatric surgeon, Dr. Miles, relayed to me that I could expect to lose about 75 percent of my excess body weight. My personal weight loss included significant drops in the beginning. In the first three months after surgery, I was losing about five pounds a week. After the first five months, my weight loss each month slowed by half, although at this point I had lost 100 pounds. My personal overall average weight loss dropped as the second year approached although I continued to lose weight for two years.

Understanding Plateaus

This weight loss window begins to close for several reasons:

- The more we weigh the faster we lose because we burn more calories.
- The pouch and opening to the intestine can stretch, which means not only can we eat more food, but also the

> Even as weight loss slows, with diligent compliance to diet and exercise, we can continue to lose weight and move toward our goal weight.

food empties from the pouch sooner leaving us hungry.

- We have to work harder at losing, and since we look and feel better, our motivation to work harder may diminish.
- We tend to let old habits creep back in to our routine.

Weight loss is influenced by more than our diet, what we eat, or even what we don't eat. It is also influenced by our weight, muscle mass, metabolic rate, activity level, and compliance.

The profound weight loss that occurs after bariatric surgery is due to the intake of fewer calories than the body needs each day. Fat tissue must be burned to offset the deficit, and weight loss results.

The more we weigh, the more the weight of our body assists us in losing the weight. As our body becomes smaller, its energy requirements are decreased and our calorie requirements also become smaller. Unfortunately, this is when it becomes possible to eat more food. When the energy consumed is equal to the calories eaten, weight loss will stop or plateau. So, physically, as you near your goal, weight loss slows and eventually stops.

The experts tell us (experts are the people who understand the body better than you and I) that our body always put self-preservation first. They tell us that our body will do anything and everything in its power not to let us die from starvation. Well, I'm glad someone understands it. If this is true, then when we go on a diet, or in our case, cut our portion sizes, our body begins to slow down the rate at which we burn fuel and starts to conserve energy. Even though losing weight after surgery is faster and offers us a better chance to lose more weight than what we can lose on our own, keep in mind that our body's natural inclination is to prevent starvation. This will result in periods of plateaus.

Plateau Solutions

Yes, there are solutions. Actually, we have several options. We could try screaming at the scale (which we all have done).

Or we could get depressed and have a pity party—I'm good

> Not only is the weight not going to come off fast enough but the mental and emotional transformations take considerably longer.

at throwing parties.

Or, maybe we need to find a way to communicate to our body that it's not starving and that it's okay to let go of a few more pounds.

That sounds like a better plan. It can be as simple as changing our normal routine, diet, or activity level.

Here are a few tips I've found to help our body break through the plateau and start losing again.

- Strength training. Lifting weights and working your muscles will help to strengthen bones, increase lean muscle mass, and ultimately boost your metabolic rate.
- Vary your exercise and activity routine. If you walk a lot, then try jogging, swimming, or cycling—anything that will change the way your body is working. If you are doing low-intensity cardio work, then try some high-intensity exercise. You could also increase the length of your activity or vary your daily routine.
- Up the protein and fiber. Getting in enough protein is important for speeding up weight loss. Fiber helps keep you fuller longer, so you eat less. Remember, to eat small, frequent, and healthy meals.

Dealing with these changes in the physical is one thing, but I began to find out at this stage of the journey, just how important mindset changes would become.

Not only is the weight not going to come off fast enough but the mental and emotional transformations take considerably longer. Just like traveling to that a long-awaited destination, this trip seems much longer than it really is. Actually, the weight comes off faster than your mind and your skin can keep up with. And of course, if indeed your brain has never been invited to come along in the first place, it's probably still sitting on the porch steps—sulking. So among all the baggage of desperation, discouragement, despair, and unrealistic expectations, let us now add a travel case full of impatience.

It is important to ask ourselves how we will emotionally handle these fluctuations and plateaus. Here are a few things I found helpful.

Embrace the Process

Part of the process is to recognize these phases and be ready to make necessary adjustments as you go. It is important not to get discouraged by the emotional ups and downs of plateaus or even small gains. Even though this experience can be a wild emotional roller-coaster ride with periods of devastating stand-stills, slow inching forward, and even occasional inclines, it usually ends with fast-paced drops as we make our progression toward our goal. I found that learning to accept a few plateaus, even weight regains here and there, and keeping a positive and realistic mindset was an important part of the experience. Accepting the excitement as well as these challenging transitional changes will allow us to create a new life during our quest for long-term success.

Focus on the Process

Hang in there and be diligent. Even though this entire experience will consist of constant change, you will drop the weight. This rest will offer you a good opportunity to review your guidelines and make sure you are doing everything that is within your control, the rest will happen in time. Assess your eating habits to make sure you have not let any old unwanted eating habits creep back up. Assess your lifestyle routines, making sure you are increasing your activity and exercise. This day-to-day process requires time, diligence, and consistency to adopt new changes for a lifetime.

Examine Your Beliefs

Even though it is a good idea to examine your routine, it will also require some inward reflection. I found that is was extremely helpful to discover what I believed about this experience and who I was in light of it. There is nothing to fear. Plateaus and small weight regains don't mean there has been a failure on our part nor does it suggest that we are a failure. Remember this is a normal part of the process.

Focus on Your Overall Progress

Progress happens slowly over time and it is not always fast or measured by the scale. Use this time to celebrate your progress and your accomplishments, turning this experience into an opportunity for growth. I found it extremely helpful to refocus my mindset on the positive and what I was gaining in the process. Each day holds a new beginning.

I often think of the observation my younger son made when he was about eight years old, while practicing reading. We found some books that captivated his interest (if there were such a thing as little boys liking books at that age). He made an announcement that these particular books were his favorite. When I asked him why, he relayed a profound observation. "*Because,*" he declared, "*there is a period at the end of every page.*"

As many times as we read the books, I had never noticed. It may have been a little tiny dot, but to him, it was huge.

That little period meant that when he reached the end of every page, he had a new opportunity—a chance to pause, to reflect, and consider his position. It promised that each page would have an end, and each new page—a new beginning. What a comfort.

So it is with our weight loss experience. The story in the middle might entail some scary stuff. You could face thrilling adventures or even disappointments. But, at the end of the day, it is finished, it's behind us and tomorrow is a new day.

These are opportunities to pause and reflect on all that we have accomplished and ponder the new experiences life has to offer. Even the most seemingly insignificant things will probably be your most magnificent milestones. Record these moments and celebrations in your journal. Your body is taking a much-deserved rest and these times can give you a chance to mentally re-charge for next step in the journey.

Just around the corner will be a new page of life. It will be filled with a new opportunity, a new beginning, and a new *you* just waiting to be. And there will always be a place to pause and celebrate.

Soon you will be done with the weight loss experience and your weight will plateau for the long-run. Knowing how to manage these new changes and learning new lifestyle skills will be necessary in order to successfully unite the *"new you"* on the inside with the *"new you"* on the outside.

Plastic Surgery: Adjusting the New Me

Although, my weight loss began to slow, I was still losing weight. I was enjoying the rewards and physical freedoms that resulted from compliance. By the time I had lost 140 pounds, I was able to wear a regular size 12. Ann Taylor here I come! I was resuming normal everyday activities comfortably. I was walking three miles a day during the week and six miles a day on the weekends.

After maintaining a 150-pound loss for several months, I considered undergoing surgery to remove excess skin.

"Plastic surgery is a life-changing event." These were the first words I heard after hellos were exchanged upon my arrival in Iowa City to have the first of several cosmetic and reconstructive surgeries.

Why Iowa City?

I remember it clearly. My long-awaited issue of WLS *Lifestyles Magazine* had arrived, and I hurried to clear my schedule so that I could retreat to my favorite back porch reading spot to soak in every word. Little did I know that the words that lay printed on the pages would bring another transformation in my life.

I had subscribed to WLS *Lifestyles Magazine* early in the spring of 2006, just after gastric bypass surgery. But, for some odd reason, I had never received an issue. I kept inquiring and waiting for the bimonthly copies to arrive and ultimately I had decided that someone else must be getting my copies. But one day in the summer of 2007, my first issue arrived.

Now, I don't believe in coincidence. I had just begun consultations with several plastic surgeons in the state, including Wilmington and Charlotte. It *just so happened* that this issue had an article featuring Dr. Cram and Dr. Aly of Iowa City Plastic Surgery (ICPS) who specialized in plastic surgery for massive weight loss patients. "*I would like to have surgery here,*" I mused, thinking that it was so far out on a limb that I would surely be shot down, if not by my husband, then by the surgeon's schedule or price. Even so, my husband encouraged me to call.

A few months later, I was on a plane to Iowa City and, well, the rest is history; and "*life-changing*" was an understatement.

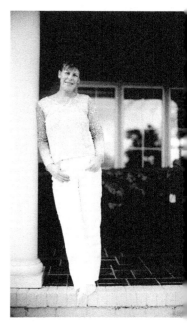

April 2008

At the time, there were no surgeons here in Wilmington performing the circumferential body lift procedure, or belt lipectomy. The surgeons in Iowa had perfected the procedure and specialized in it, along with surgical procedures for the arms and legs. A lipectomy is a whole different ball game from just getting a tummy tuck. It is a 360-degree cut, all the way around.

I wanted someone who knew the special needs that were involved for a massive weight loss patient. Dr. Aly and Cram are leaders in their field. They are in great demand all over the US and the world. Dr. Aly has written the first textbook on body contouring after massive weight loss.

The fact that they specialized in these procedures meant that I could be confident that I was receiving the best care and expertise in the field. They knew how to cater to my specific needs, including blood work, protein levels, and BMI. It is recommended that you be at your goal weight and maintaining for several months. I recommend years not just months. After you read the chapter about weight regain, you will understand why I say this. ICPS requires that you meet the criteria and your BMI is under 35. Having the surgery too soon is not advised as this will affect your results and safety.

Since I was going to invest this much money into my body, I was going for the very best I could afford. This was a decision that would affect the rest of my life.

Another factor that led to my decision to travel to Iowa City was the fact that there were two surgeons performing the operation, which reduced the time in the operating room. I stayed in the hospital for several nights, which was another deciding factor for me. In most places, you just stay one night in a surgical center with one nurse on duty. I felt that this procedure was far too extensive to be done without hospital care.

Another important advantage was the excellent pain management. I received an epidural, which helped prevent blood clots as well as pain. I was also given an internal automatic pain pump, which was activated before leaving the hospital and overlapped the epidural. In addition, I was given oral pain medication as needed.

The surgeons believe that recovering from one surgery at a time is all the body can do well, so they only perform one at a time. Undergoing multiple surgeries at once is very hard on the body and results in a slow recovery.

I was looking for a procedure that could also tighten the abdominal wall muscle without an additional incision, which ICPS could perform.

I made a quick recovery, which I believe was due, in part, to the excellent, world-class surgical and personal medical care I received through ICPS and Mercy Hospital—and also to the fact that I had been very vigilant with my protein and a healthy diet. And, of course, the "world-class" care of my husband who so graciously took care of me during my recovery. And most certainly—prayer.

Gastric bypass is life changing; but plastic surgery goes beyond the physical, beyond diet changes and exercise, even size. Plastic surgery helps you to regain your self-confidence. I don't know if I can really put into words what the surgery has done for me mentally. Iowa City Plastic Surgery says it this way: "...it eliminates forever the 'I still feel fat' feeling, giving patients the body that allows them *to enjoy their newfound health and well-being."*

I soon discovered, there was still more work to be done in the "feeling fat" department, but the reconstruction did help me look younger and move with more flexibility. It has helped restore the body I thought was lost forever. It was great to know that the surgeons I chose could relate to my specific needs and desires, understand my motivations, and assist me in determining a realistic expectation. I have been overwhelmingly pleased with the results.

I later returned to Iowa City several times, for additional surgeries including arms and legs.

No matter what decision you make, it is important to inform yourself on the procedures and qualifications of the surgeons and to have confidence in those which you choose.

PART FOUR:

Tests, Trials, and Temptations

Weight Loss Surgery Phase Four: The Post-Surgical Long-Term Maintenance Phase

People who have given up are ruled by their darkest mistakes, worst failures and deepest regrets. If you want to be successful, then be governed by your finest thoughts, your highest enthusiasm, your greatest optimism, and your most triumphant experiences.

John C. Maxwell

Mirror, Mirror: A Dream or Reality?

One cannot think crooked and walk straight.
Author Unknown

In April 2008, I celebrated my 2-year surgery anniversary with a 164-pound weight loss, a clean bill of health, 100 percent freedom from prescription and over-the-counter medications, a new (size 6) body, and a new name, "MeMe."

Finally, my dream of losing weight and regaining health had come true. I had reached my goal weight, gained health, and found a wonderfully new and exciting life. By everyone else's definition of success, I was there. I should have been in paradise. But deep down I knew there was still something missing. I had no idea what it was, but I knew I wasn't there yet.

There was a new image in the mirror, but it wasn't the same as the one in my head. I was having a huge struggle getting my head and my body on the same page.

My close friends, even family members, didn't recognize me. On one occasion, my husband "lost" me in the mall—I was standing right beside him.

At a dinner party, I bumped into someone in an attempt to maneuver around a table. As I started to apologize, I realized it wasn't another person at all. It was a mirror and the unfamiliar reflection was my own.

In the past, I had avoided mirrors and photographs, anything that would reflect my appearance. That reflection was not the real me either. Nevertheless, it was an image I lived with and accepted for years.

Now, I was spending many hours staring at my reflection in the mirror, trying to talk myself into believing that the image I saw belonged to me. I could see it was physically real, I could touch and feel it was real; but in my mind, it was not.

I was sure that the clothes that went into the dryer were smaller when they came out dry and clean. Someone surely was playing tricks on me. These couldn't be my clothes; they were too small. I must have shrunk them for sure. I would take them out of the dryer and try them on to see if I could still wear them, and to my surprise, I could.

After years of failure and low self esteem, I was very unsure of myself. I had a hard time giving myself credit for my accomplishments. I needed permission to be proud of myself without feeling prideful, arrogant, or self-centered.

Sometimes, I felt as though I was living in a dream and that at any moment I would wake up and it would all disappear. This is the entry I recorded in my journal:

I feel as though this is too good to be true and that I am going to wake up from a dream. When I see my reflection in the mirror, someone else seems to be standing in my place. I can touch it and feel it and see it, but the reality is just not there. My brain seems to be lagging somewhere behind. One day I know the reality will take me past my disbelief. Until that time, I can keep looking at my accomplishments and my old photos, recalling my recent transformations hoping that this "one day" will come soon.

CHAPTER 27

VI. Thou Shalt Establish A New Way of Thinking

**Sow a thought, reap an act,
sow an act, reap a habit,
sow a habit, reap a lifestyle,
sow a lifestyle, reap a destiny.**

Unknown Origin

During the weight loss process, our body undergoes a tremendous transformation, on the outside. Thing is, our inner selves need revision as well as our outer. We've been wearing our in side out—and it shows.

I discovered some rather cute and unusual teddy BEARS, by artist Kent Rogowski. These odd-looking bears have been turned inside out and re-stuffed. You can imagine how they look wearing their insides out. There eyes turn inward; their seams are worn outwards. They seem rather deniably unaware that their stuffing tends to spill from all directions. The creator of these bears says it is an artistic approach to offering a metaphor for us all to consider *"These bears, which have lived and loved and lost as much as their owners, have suffered and endured through it all. It is by virtue of revealing their inner core might we better understand our own."*

These BEARS look a little strange, but they are also thought provoking. It is the inward issues that trip us up, not just the physical ones. If we could see ourselves inside out, things might not look so healthy. Or maybe that is exactly what we are seeing on the outside. We let our outer shape our inner and our inner shape our outer. What we really need is to alter more than our stomachs.

Phase Four: The Long-term Maintenance Phase

Like the Israelites, I'm sure you expected that we would be in the Promised Land by now, but we're not there yet. Once we meet our weight loss goal, we pass out of the weight loss phase and enter into another: *The Long-term Maintenance Phase.* Long-term maintenance means, well, long-term. So, as bariatric patients, we are also reaching the longest leg of our journey.

Learning to become skilled in maintenance takes time and practice. Long-term maintenance is an ongoing process that will allow us to discover our new normal. Since we will be living in this phase for a while, it will also be important for us to make the best of our time here. After all, this is a new place and a new experience for us and we will need to learn how to hold on to our weight loss success in order to be successful for the long haul.

During our weight loss phase we have experienced radical weight loss as well as vivid outward changes. Here in this phase however, our weight loss has stopped and there are no obvious miracles taking place. It all seems to have come to a standstill. In this phase, it is very easy to overlook our progress. If we're not careful, our entire weight loss experience can become distorted and out of focus. It may seem as though we are not making forward progress, walking in circles, destined to repeat our past. We can easily become frustrated and disillusioned with the entire experience.

If there is one thing that I began to understand along the way, it was that my efforts needed to be equally focused on the journey and the process it took to reach the destination, as much as on the end result.

Even though it seemed that nothing was happening on the surface, there were indeed tremendous transformations taking place within.

> **If there is one thing that I began to understand along the way, it was that my efforts needed to be equally focused on the journey and the process it took to reach the destination, as much as on the end result.**

Little By Little

There is a verse from the book of *Exodus*. It became a familiar verse that had been playing over and over in my mind. *"Little by little I will drive them (your enemies) out before you, until you have increased enough to take possession of the land." Exodus 23:30*

My journey over the past two years had been all about decreasing, but suddenly the word "increase" seemed to strangely consume my thoughts. Increase? Would I need to *increase* in order to take possession of my land? If possession required increase, what was "increase" about? How much increasing must I do? What would possession of the land look like in my everyday life? Would there be enemies that would keep me from holding on to my hard earned success? What next?

After months of pondering this verse, and going back to study it again and again, I realized that there was indeed a principal for weight loss success within those words.

The disciplines I had built of wiser choices and lifestyle changes had come little by little, but I found I had much more to learn about how to maintain weight loss.

In order to get my mind and body on the same page, I had more enemies to fight and some more overcoming to do.

Yes, the pounds were gone, but the diet mentality, the body image, and the possibility of weight regain were not. I had to learn to keep the weight off. This was a new challenge in and of itself and it was one in which I had little to no experience.

I was still experiencing emotional episodes that drew me towards food. There were times I would find myself in the pantry when I knew I shouldn't be eating. I had to continue to focus on the increase of positive behavioral changes to hold on to the success I had earned.

There was still something missing, and I was determined to find it. The Promised Land was out there somewhere and I needed to possess it—whatever that meant. I set my mind to increasing. As the days and months ticked by, I trusted that little by little, day by day would bring me closer, until I had increased—enough.

What's Next, Brain Surgery?

The physical weight was gone and I had gained physical health, but there were still things that were holding me back—a struggle between the inner and the outer. I began to change my focus from the external weight loss to the progression of another sort—the internal experience.

Let's see—stomach surgery, reconstructive surgery. What's next, brain surgery? Well, this is where brain surgery would help if it were that simple, but I am certain it requires a bit more than that. Weight loss surgery isn't brain surgery, but that's exactly what we need. But not the kind we can get from a hospital or a physical operating room with carbon steel scalpels, stainless steel staples, and silicone bands. Neither does it require professional surgeons or leaders in the field of bariatrics, psychology, or neurology. It is not just what we *do* that shapes us, it's what we *think*. Believe it or not, the gateway to change is through our thoughts.

It is not just what we *do* that shapes us, it's what we *think*.

If you remember in the pre-surgery stage, we talked about mindset changes and how important they were. It wasn't until after I had gastric bypass surgery that I really began to understand how essential it would be to examine my thoughts and beliefs. At this point, my inward issues were still making themselves evident on the outside.

There is a new technique now being performed called Gastric Mind Banding Surgery. The professionals who administer it call it surgery but it's actually hypnosis. Hypnosis is based on the power of the mind and a heightened susceptibility to suggestion. They suggest to people under hypnosis that they have had weight loss surgery. I'm **not** suggesting that you have hypnosis. However, it does have a high measure of success, which suggests that what we think has a great impact on how we act and how we live out our lives. What we think affects us more than we know.

In her book, *Who Switched Off My Brain*, researcher Dr. Caroline Leaf has scientifically determined that thoughts and emotions affect our body. Toxic thoughts undermine and destroy our immune system, preventing its ability to do what it was designed to do. She also explains research which shows around 87 percent of illnesses can be attributed to our thought life, and approximately 13 percent to diet, genetics, and environment. Studies conclusively link many chronic diseases to an epidemic of toxic emotions in our culture.

There is no longer any doubt that what we think affects our emotional and physical state. I am convinced that our thought process can work with us or against us in our effort toward reaching and sustaining weight loss success.

Actually this information is not as new as it seems. The bible has much to say about the way our thinking can affect us. True transformation takes place in the mind. Who we are is determined by what we think.

Between 450-350 BC, Hippocrates, The Father of Medicine believed, *"Illness occurs when the body's systems are toxic and out-of-balance. One must treat the body as a whole, rather than a series of parts."*

We are not just a series of unrelated parts and we are not just physical beings. We can't just fix our outer physical selves and not change our inner selves. We have several dimensions; we have a body, a soul, and a spirit. These three aspects work together. As a matter a fact, they are so intricately woven together that what affects one, affects the other.

Our soul is made up of three aspects as well.

- *Our mind* (our thinker)
- *Our emotions* (our feeler)
- *Our will* (our chooser)

Understanding how these aspects of our makeup work will help us to understand why we can't just address obesity from the physical aspect alone. We must also look at our mindset and how it affects us as a whole. In the next few chapters, I will share with you how these mindset changes became an important part of my success.

Romans 12:2

... be transformed by the renewing of your mind ...

(NKJV)

My intention is to give you a simple overview, from my research, combined with my personal experience, so that you can understand why our thoughts are important and how they shape our lives. When we understand our belief system and how it is formed, we can change how we respond and how we live.

When we are presented with a thought, we choose whether to believe it. These thoughts influence and establish our belief system. What we choose to believe becomes our perception.

Our perceptions become our truth and our reality. This is why two people can experience the same event and have very different views. What we perceive *feels* true to *us*. We feel what we believe. In other words, a belief is always attached to a feeling. Then, we respond or act based on how we feel.

These beliefs are called *core beliefs* and they are based on our perception of truth about ourselves and the world around us.

Our beliefs affect our self-worth, our self-esteem, and our self-image. They become our identity. Our identity doesn't just come from what we see in the mirror or our physical reality. Our identity goes much deeper. These beliefs are formed by:

- How we see ourselves.
- How we perceive others see us.
- How we view our world.

These core beliefs begin to form early in our lives. Most professionals agree that these core beliefs are set by the time we reach early adolescences. Before we are old enough to decide our own standard, our standards are imposed by others.

In an effort to discover what motivated me to act, I began to revisit my core beliefs. Only then could I get to the root of what I believed and why I believed it. It helped me to determine why I felt what I felt, and why I did what I did.

My journey was about finding truth. I had to learn to identify destructive lies, or past perceptions no longer relevant, tear them down, and replace them with new present truths.

Therefore, we must take a look at what we believe about ourselves. Neither dieting, exercise, hypnotic suggestion, nor weight loss surgery can offer us *total* solutions to freedom from obesity. I'm not saying they don't work, they do. But we can't stop there. We can't just address the physical aspect and not the rest of us.

It may serve, to some degree, as a convincing measure to just believe that you have had lap-band or gastric bypass surgery, but that puts us right back in the same sinking ship. Changing our *behavior* alone does not solve the deeper issue. You can out-eat *mind* surgery, just as you can out-eat the real surgery.

I believe our freedom starts with taking a serious look at our core beliefs and the things that directly influence our feelings and our choices. Weight loss surgery changed my body, but I had to change my thoughts. I had to uncover the *root causes* that were keeping me from success.

I don't know about you, but I'm not looking for mind banding; and neither do I want to be ruled by my emotions. I'm looking for mind freedom. Mind freedom includes emotional freedom. Emotional freedom comes from discovering truth.

The emotional freedom I was looking for required a desire to explore what brought me to this intersection in my life so that I wouldn't end up back in obesity again. I needed to find out *why* I ate. I needed to get past the surface reactions and go to the core root of *what was eating me*. As I began to examine my thoughts and my core beliefs, I was able to make the necessary changes. Finding truth allowed me to step into a new place of freedom that went beyond the physical.

When I discovered the truth, the truth set me free. A change of mind and thought was a huge step toward healing and recovery. These changes affected my entire life and allowed me to go forward into success.

This process takes determination and commitment. It is not the *"easy way out,"* but, for me, it was the *"real way out."*

It can be for you, too. Your new reality is just a thought away.

CHAPTER 28

VII. Thou Shalt No Longer Use False Labels And Negative Self Talk

As a man thinks in his heart, so is he.

Proverbs 23:7

What happens next in the story of the Israelites is a perfect illustration of how our thoughts can hold us back from moving forward in our search for success.

Back at the campground, the Israelites were making preparations to leave the desert and enter into the land of promise. It is apparent that their expectation was to go in immediately without hesitation, *"thinking it easy" (Deuteronomy 1:41)* to conquer the enemy and take back their land.

Never having been there before, a decision was made to send a few scouts ahead into the land to investigate the territory: to identify what lay within its boundaries and to bring back some of the fruit of the land. Moses selected 12 leaders from among the people. These scouts left their family tribes and set out to explore the land of their dreams.

At the end of 40 days, they brought back an account for the whole assembly. Two, of the leaders, Joshua and Caleb, reported that the land was a good land. The people who lived there were strong and the cities were large and well fortified. Described as a land flowing with milk and honey, it was just as God had promised. It was a picture of agricultural abundance with fertile soil, brooks, springs, and plentiful crops. In fact, the fruit was so extravagant, it took two men to carry one single cluster of grapes back to camp.

Joshua and Caleb wholeheartedly expressed their faith that the Lord had given them the land. They encouraged the Israelites to not be afraid. They inspired them to be strong and courageous, to fight for what was rightfully theirs, for they were well able to possess it.

However, the other ten scouts who went into the land had a different perspective and they told a different version of what they believed about what they saw. "*We can't attack those people, they are stronger than we are. The land we explored devours those living in it. All the people we saw were of great size. We seemed like grasshoppers in our own eyes, and we looked the same to them.*" (Numbers 13:31,32,33)

All of the men had gone in together, and they all saw the same things. But their reports were extremely different. Their versions of what they believed about what they had seen had conflicting details. How could this be? Why did they have different accounts?

During the journey, Joshua had become a proven military leader. In *Numbers 13*, the biblical account tells us that Moses changed Joshua's name, a sign that he has accepted his new identity. Joshua and Caleb had totally and wholeheartedly chosen to believe that God had given them the land and they saw themselves as strong and well able to go in and take it. They had chosen to accept their new reality. The difference between Joshua and Caleb and the others was their *perspective* or their *perception*.

When the Israelites were in Egypt they were surrounded by a tangible enemy—one they could see. When they crossed the Red Sea, they thought they had left the enemy far behind them. But now as they prepared to go into the land, they discovered that there was another enemy before them. Not only the people that dwelled in the land must be overcome, but there was also an enemy that was *unseen*—one that was within them.

The Israelites had been slaves for a very long time. Their situation had changed. Except for Joshua and Caleb, their perception of how they saw themselves had not. Their truth had been based on who they were in the past—a former truth.

They were still using their old labels. In their minds they saw themselves as *"grasshoppers"*—small, weak, and insignificant, not military conquerors, or land owners. They also perceived that this was the way they looked to their enemies. Even after seeing the tangible evidence of the fruit of the land for themselves, the entire assembly agreed with the negative report.

What they needed was a new identity. Possession of the land must be built on their present truth. They were no longer slaves. They were landowners. It would be necessary to establish a new image of themselves. Their present identity needed to match their present reality.

Giant Sized Perceptions

It seems that once out of slavery, it was a simple matter of letting go of who they were in the past and embrace their new reality. But, I can tell you; it's not that simple. Once out of obesity, I found it wasn't simple for me, either.

Getting used to a new body image was a big adjustment. As my body rapidly tried to adjust to massive weight loss, my mind was finding it hard to keep up. My body was saying one thing and my mind was saying another. My own conflicting report was holding me back from entering into my new land.

Sometimes it is hard to break away from the things that hold us in the past. This process takes time, it doesn't just happen overnight, nor does it happen all by itself.

Did you ever wonder how an elephant could be trained or held in captivity, since it could so easily break free from the chains that hold it? Elephants are one of the largest, strongest, and smartest animals that live on land. They have been trained to lift heavy loads for thousands of years and they can carry over 600 pounds and can move heavy objects that weigh in excess of two tons. Yet it only takes a small chain to hold them.

It all starts when the elephants are young and relatively weak. When training elephants, keepers chain a leg of very small

Sometimes it is hard to break away from the things that hold us in the past. This process takes time, it doesn't just happen overnight, nor does it happen all by itself.

elephant to a huge, heavy chain connected to a deeply driven peg. The small elephant learns it is useless to try to break away.

As the elephant grows, keepers use the same shackle but with a smaller and smaller chain attached to a shallower and shallower peg. The keepers no longer need the heavy chain or the deep peg. The elephant has learned that it is senseless to fight against it. The shackles still yield the same results for the 10,000-pound elephant that could easily walk away with the chain, the peg, and the keepers, too.

The elephant has the strength to do what ever it wants, but its mind does not have the same message because there is a conflicting report. The reality has changed, but their perception of the situation has not. Everyone knows that the elephant has the strength to break away—except the elephant. It's not the chain that holds the adult elephant. It's what the elephant believes. The elephant still carries the belief that he does not possess the strength or the power to break the ties that hold him in captivity.

I realized that if I didn't get my mind and my body on the same track, the physical reality would slip right through my fingers and that, one day, I just might wake up to the reality that was still inside my head. This image was not the one in the mirror; it was still the 300-pound girl I thought I left behind.

New Body, New Image

Several months went by and I began taking a class to get my certification as a bariatric coach. We were learning about core beliefs. During one of the sessions I suddenly realized what was keeping me from making the mind-body connection.

I discovered it is possible to hold two conflicting beliefs at the same time and I realized that my struggle was based on two conflicting reports.

I once *was* obese. That fact *was* true. However, physically I had changed. This was also true. I could see and feel the reality. But somewhere inside I was also *believing* I was the same old me. I had still been holding on to the old image of myself. I had told myself repeatedly for years that I was hopelessly overweight, that things were never going to change, and I would always be overweight and unhealthy. This was my core belief.

That is when the light came on. Yes, I once was stuck in that body, but not anymore. The belief that I would never change was no longer true. I was believing a lie. The circumstances had changed. I had changed. I was different. I had been holding on to an old label that was no longer relevant. I had to let go of my 300-pound label.

It sounds so simple, but I was holding two beliefs, and the old one was ruling over the new one. These two conflicting reports had created a *disconnect*. The old truth had not allowed me to "see" my true size. One truth had to dominate. I had to make a choice to believe the new truth and to discard the old one. That simple insight unlocked my mind. It immediately put my mind and body on the same page.

Replacing the old beliefs took more than trying on clothes, or standing in front of the mirror, or even the long talks I had with myself, in hopes that one day it would be real.

I'll give you the steps again.

- I had to examine and identify my core belief.
- I asked myself if that belief was the present truth.
- This allowed me to make a choice. I had to decide which truth I would embrace, the old perception of truth or the new present reality.
- Once I recognized the lie, I made a choice to replace it with the new truth.
- When I agreed with the new truth, I began see the image of myself the way I was, in the present.

Getting my mind and body on the same page was a huge milestone in my journey. From this point on, the focus of my journey became to find truth. I had to learn to identify and tear down false perceptions, destructive lies, past truths no longer relevant, and old labels that held me in the past and replace them with the new truths of the present.

What Not to Wear: Old Labels

We are all familiar with labels. We use labels as a unit of measure. We use them to assign our limits. After weight loss surgery, it is important to establish limits. Some limits are useful, especially when it comes to our new diet. But have you ever thought about the labels that we apply to ourselves? Our internal labels also set our limits. Our old labels keep us tied to our old self-image and can limit our potential. In order to change our outward actions, we must go beyond what we believe about our *circumstances*, and we must also take a look at what we believe about *ourselves*.

I began reading a book by John Maxwell, *The Difference Maker*. There was a question in the book that I began to give serious consideration. *"Do you believe you are a highly competent and successful person who sometimes fails, or are you basically a failure who is working to avoid mistakes?"* "Ouch." As Curly of the Three Stooges would say, *"I resemble that remark!"*

Let's read that statement again, but this time, make it personal. *"Do I believe I am a highly competent and successful person who sometimes fails, or am I basically a failure who is working to avoid mistakes?"*

This is where my journey led me down a different path toward a more inward focus. I began to take a good, hard look at the other labels I had placed on myself.

How do we see ourselves? What do we believe about ourselves? After losing weight, we become a new person on the outside, but if we haven't changed on the inside, we may need a new identity and a new label.

One of the first things we change after weight loss is our clothing size. It is an exciting time. However, shopping for clothing was probably one of the hardest things I had to do after losing weight. I had no idea how to dress myself. I wasn't familiar with current clothing styles. But, it wasn't just about my outward

> Our old labels keep us tied to our old self-image and can limit our potential.

appearance. Recovering from obesity is not just about wearing a new physical body and it means more than getting to wear new, smaller, stylish outer clothing. It's not just about what we wear, it's about what *not* to wear—old labels. We can't hold on to our old identity any more than we can keep wearing our old size clothing.

Whether it's the teenager in a self-discovery phase, the preppy college student, or diligent homemaker, what we choose to wear reflects how we see ourselves—that is, unless we are obese. When I was obese, I had just one shopping rule: if it fit my body and somewhat hid the fat bulges, I purchased it.

The larger sized clothes I purchased were nice (XXX-tra nice, and expensive) but the cuts were limited and unstylish. They didn't express my personality. Those former 3-X sizes weren't the least bit youthful. I really felt more like a 90-year-old, and that is the way I saw myself: old. Even though deep down somewhere I wanted to feel young, it was buried very deep.

After losing weight, I remember asking my friend, La Cretia, if the blouse I was wearing was too tight. She said something that remains with me even today. She looked me straight in the eye and said, "*It's fine, and you don't have to hide anymore.*" I found I had to lose more than physical weight. I had to lose the heavy emotional weight that I had been carrying around. The big, bulky clothes did more than just cover my body. They actually hid me. I hid behind self-doubt, low self-worth, depleted self-esteem, and a poor self-image.

I struggled with letting go of the old clothes. You know, just in case the surgery didn't work. After countless diets, failure was common. This was a brand new experience, and I had to bring my mind along to the present. I quickly realized that I had to let go of the old label that said I was a failure at losing weight and keeping it off. I knew if I kept hanging on to those old clothes, they would serve as a crutch to fall back on. I had to give up all of that X-size clothing and along with them I needed to find new positive labels. I needed to start revealing the new me. However, I had no idea who I really was.

> We can't hold on to our old identity any more than we can keep wearing our old size clothing.

There were many conflicting reports. One part of me wanted to reveal my personality and increasing sense of self-worth and confidence. On the other hand, I was unprepared and unsure how I felt about exposing my true self.

Who Am I?

As I tried on clothing, it was like searching for clues about who I was under all that emotional clutter. I was sometimes surprised by the style of clothing that appealed to me and wondered what new emotions were being revealed that I had hidden away for so long. Was I choosing clothes that reflected my new identity and personality?

I wondered if the clothes I liked were "age appropriate." I had to keep reminding myself that I was 50 now. I would ask the attendants in the clothing store, if it were age appropriate and how old they thought I was. But I never got an answer. I soon realized, these were things I would have to discover on my own. I had to learn to take responsibility for my success. I couldn't hide behind excuses any longer.

I was having to discover who I was and what statement I really wanted to make. I was beginning to realize that the old image of myself just didn't fit within the margins of the new "me" anymore. I knew it would be up to me to examine my inner beliefs and to find out what other adjustments had to be made to bring my "inward" into alignment with my "outward".

I found I had to lose all the years of accumulated criticisms, prejudices, stereotypes, and perceptions of how I saw myself, how others saw me, and I how I viewed the world around me. Some of these old images had been growing for a long time. Some were very deep rooted and took much longer to uproot than others.

I found that some of these thoughts have been driven very deep within my mind and spirit. These old labels didn't just start when I started to gain weight or after I became obese. I found that I had been carrying old labels around since childhood.

These old labels started to form early in my life. Some formed from simple or seemingly insignificant events and others from traumatic experiences in my past.

One such incident occurred when I was in the second grade. I was accused by my teacher of something I did not do. I was called up in front of the class and in front of everyone I was accused of cheating and I was slapped in the face. I was not given a chance to offer an explanation, or defend myself. I was embarrassed, humiliated, and physically hurt. I was alone and wounded.

These beliefs were embedded with emotions and resulted in how I felt. I felt devalued and shamed. I felt helpless to plead my case. I felt insignificant and unimportant. I felt trapped and unprotected.

Afterwards other moments in my life triggered those painful memories and offered me countless opportunities to replay these thoughts in my head. Coming into agreement with them, these thoughts became my *perception* of truth and formed my core beliefs.

Other life situations that followed also became triggers that brought me back to that same conclusion. Much later in life these same feelings cropped up whenever I was in a situation in which I had no control, was misjudged, wrongly accused, mistrusted, and unable to express my intentions or give an explanation for my actions.

Each time I agreed with these beliefs, thoughts and feelings, these beliefs began to form into an identity. I am unloved and uncared for. I am not trustworthy. I am not important. I am uniquely flawed. I am a bad person. I am stupid. I am hopeless and helpless. I am not worthy of being heard. I am alone and wounded.

I thought, I believed, I felt, I became.

These emotional traumas form shameful scars and leave us to suffer in silence. We are held in the suffocating grip of captivity, depression, and self-condemnation. As we rehearse these defeating thoughts over and over we are held in an emotional prison and we are convinced there is no way of escape.

So, is it any wonder we have found eating as a means to cover up, soothe, or escape old hurts and wounds of the past? Is it any wonder that after years of being overweight and an endless stream of failures that we see ourselves as powerless to break free from the old images of how we see ourselves? Is it any wonder that even after massive weight loss, we don't know who we are?

Getting To Know The New Me

As I began to uproot the negative beliefs I held about who I was, I discovered how much power I did have to break away from the invisible chains that were holding me captive. Part of the process involved listening to what I was saying to myself.

Strange thought, isn't it? Listening to yourself. In any relationship, communication is foundational, it's the way we get to know each other, and I needed to get to know myself. I knew the old me pretty well, but I needed a new image of the new me. I needed to re-image.

Reimage is a computer term. Reimage is the process of removing all the old software on a computer and reinstalling everything. A reimage is necessary if your operating system becomes damaged or corrupted. And that is exactly what I needed to do. It was time to reimage.

It was also time for the Olympic games to begin and I had been seen running around the house with a 2-year-old. No, not AFTER a 2-year-old, WITH a 2-year-old! Gavin and I have invented a few games of our own. We defined our starting line and readied ourselves for the countdown. 1...2...3...ready...set...go! Then it was off to the races. Down the hall, through the foyer and maybe even a detour through the kitchen.

This game required socks. Slippery ones. Papa's weren't the right kind. But, for Gavin and MeMe, we had just the right slickness to slip and slide without falling down.

As we slid across the finish line, Gavin would pause in wonder that his grandmother was allowing him to run in the house. And, not only that, she was leading in the excitement. To a 2 ½ year-old little boy, what could be more fun?

I will admit, it sounds more like child's play than the Olympics.

Before weight loss, I couldn't have kept up with a 2-year-old. I wouldn't have been doing much running, and I certainly wouldn't have been sliding in stocking feet through the house. Before weight loss, I could only dream.

What, then, is this race all about? For those in the Olympics, it's for the gold. I'm sure they all have different reasons for their passion. For Gavin this race was just about the fun. For me, however, it was more about the relationship I shared with my first grandchild.

I'm very thankful for the time I have to spend with him. Building the relationship is priceless and it gives me the wonderful opportunity to watch his character develop and grow. As Gavin and I build a relationship we are *both* discovering our new personalities beginning to emerge.

In the past, I really had not given any thought to building a healthy relationship with *myself*. As a matter of fact, I didn't even know I had a relationship with myself. It was a discovery that became a priority.

We spend time with ourselves constantly. As a matter of fact, we can't get away from ourselves. We are in constant communication. We talk to ourselves all the time. Talking to ourselves doesn't mean we're crazy. It is something we all do, even if we aren't always aware of it.

This is referred to as our *self-talk*. It's what we are saying to ourselves that is important. This internal coach, can encourage us, boost our confidence, and motivate us to achieve our goals; or it can be like an internal tyrant, undermining, criticizing, and beating us up.

Q What are we saying to ourselves?

Q Do we display the type of person we want to be, towards ourselves?

Q Are we kind?

Q Do we build ourselves up or tear ourselves down?

Q Do we encourage ourselves or throw ourselves under the bus?

Q Do we value, care for, appreciate, or even love ourselves?

Gold medal winners don't accomplish the goal or even go through the motions by telling themselves they can't or that they are no good. They are winners because they tell themselves they are winners, they see themselves as winners, and their actions are based on what they think and believe.

It took time and practice to identify my old thinking patterns and replace them with new positive self-talk. It was a method of increasing—an increase in my self-worth, my self-esteem, a new self-image, and a new identity—even so, there was even more to come.

News From the Dryer

The increase I needed was indeed, little by little. I was always amazed when I could do things with such ease because, in my mind, they still seemed difficult or even impossible. It took several years before I didn't hesitate before reaching down for things on the floor, especially if I was seated. Even now, I am still discovering all the things I can do that I couldn't do before losing weight.

I am continually reminded of how I can put on tights with great ease, and I can wear panty hose again—just because I can. Neither do they cut off the circulation of my legs nor do I punch holes with every pull because they actually move upward without delay.

I can even wear shoes with strings (because I can tie them myself). I can put on boots without a struggle. I can bend at the hip, slide my foot into my boot, and get back up again—all while breathing, without fainting or turning red in the face. When I return to a standing position, my pants aren't ripped in the seat, either. Amazing! And the other foot goes in just as easily. Imagine that. But, I don't just have to imagine it. I'm doing it.

Remember the song, "These Boots Are Made for Walking" and the line "one of these days these boots are going to walk all over you." That is just about how I felt before losing weight. The boots, and even shoes for that matter, had already won the battle before ever making it onto my feet. Not anymore. Now, I love wearing boots. Yep, these boots are made for walking, and that's just what I'm doing.

Funny, we weight loss surgery patients appreciate things most people take for granted. After massive weight loss, doing everyday things takes on a different perspective. Massive weight loss. That still has a funny ring to it. Who me? Massive weight loss?

There were times, especially after I started wearing smaller size clothes, that I was hesitant to put them in the dryer. Before surgery, I would never put my clothes in the dryer. However, as my clothes got roomier, I began to put them into the dryer to shrink them on purpose. What a concept.

Not only am I different on the outside, I'm different on the inside. It just occurred to me one day as I did the laundry, that I could, without a second thought, take my clothes from the washer to the dryer, set the timer, and push the button. I retrieve the clothes from the dryer and hang them on their hangers. It doesn't even occur to me any longer to try them on or even question the fact that I can still wear them. They belong to me. Of course, they fit. I now have established ownership of my new body image.

Finding truth set me free. Bringing my false beliefs into the light of real truth, and learning how to tear down the lies that bound me, allowed me to find freedom.

There was more healing to come and many tremendously important life-changing truths to discover. I started to focus on the miracles that were happening everyday.

Raindrops On Noses

There are so many unique adventures that MeMe's and their grandchildren can create together. There was the day Gavin and I planned an exciting trip to the bookstore. We hunted for the best book ever, played with the Thomas train set, and then headed for lunch.

Of course, mealtime with a toddler is always an adventure. After playing in the play area for a while, it was time to head home

> Bringing my false beliefs into the light of real truth, and learning how to tear down the lies that bound me, allowed me to find freedom.

for a much-needed break for MeMe and a nap for Gavin. That was when I noticed that what I thought was a passing shower of sprinkling raindrops had become a full-fledged rainstorm, and it was coming down by the bucket loads. With both arms full of cups, bags, and one adorable little boy, I didn't have an extra hand for an umbrella. At the first sign of a let up, we braved the rain and headed to the car between drops.

Of course, I had parked at the far end of the parking lot, and as we neared the car the rain resumed even harder than before. By the time I got the car door open, my only option, rather than drowning, was to dart into the back seat.

I managed to buckle Gavin in while standing up in the car and leaning over the car seat. Gavin, meanwhile, pointed out the fact that we were soaked. After taking a few minutes to collect myself and then drying us off a bit, I began to think of what my next option might be for getting to the driver's seat. A quick look outside at the downpour left me with only one choice, the unthinkable. Yes, I did! I actually crawled and maneuvered over the seat and into the front! I did it, and as I was bringing my contorted limbs over the seat, I realized that this event would never have happened several years before.

Yes, we were both wet, but laughing at ourselves as water drops came trickling down our noses. What a fun time—a little more exercise than I anticipated, but nevertheless, I was thrilled just to be able to do it.

Three years earlier, I would not have been able to run across the parking lot with a toddler in tow, climb in the backseat of the car head first with a kid in my arms (a rather smooth and quick move, I must say), stand up in the back seat (managing a child, which is a feat in and of itself), nor even think about climbing into the front seat from the back.

It's the change in thinking that transforms the most ordinary, mundane, and everyday moments into extra-ordinary, super-fabulous, and wonder-filled adventures. Thanks, Gavin, for helping MeMe feel young. And thank You, God, for raindrop moments. I hope this part never changes.

CHAPTER 29

VIII. Thou Shalt Remember Thy Past, But Not Dwell There

Those who can't remember the past are condemned to repeat it.

Philosopher George Santayana

More than five hundred years earlier God had made a promise to Abraham to give him and his descendants an inheritance. God kept His promise. He has delivered Abraham's descendants out of Egypt. But remember, just because they are out of Egypt, doesn't mean Egypt is out of them.

When we last left the Israelites, they had just gotten a glimpse of the Promised Land before them. God had promised to go before them and drive out the inhabitants that dwelled in the land. In order to possess the land, they needed to be strong and courageous and go in and take it. But they struggled to let go of their old mindsets. They were landowners, but they still viewed themselves as slaves—weak and vulnerable. Even with God's help, they feared the new territory would devour them and they would not be able to overcome the seemingly giant-sized obstacles that lay before them. This conflicting report was causing some major conflicts.

Not only did these beliefs delay their progress, but they also robbed them of their ability to live in the Promised Land. Because of their unwillingness to let go of these old beliefs, God declared that they could not move on until the entire doubting generation and their old mindsets were eliminated. God told the Israelites that they would spend the next 40 years in the desert.

Before they were just passing through this desert, but now they must live there—wandering. What began as an eleven-day hike had then stretched into a forty-year journey.

From reading the passages in scripture there isn't much recorded about their time in the desert, except that they moved around and around in a circle for 40 years. Therefore, it's easy to assume that they weren't making any progress. But even though they literally wandered in circles for years, each lap around the desert was another lap toward their ultimate victory.

A 40-year sentence may feel like a severe punishment, but they had some "baggage" to unload. No longer slaves, they needed a new identity before they could be successful in a new land. But they didn't just need a new identity, they had some other mentalities to unload. It takes time to discard old mindsets and 40 years is certainty a long time. In the bible, the number "40" symbolizes a time of probation, testing, or trial. This 40-year time frame will allow them time to let go of the old. It will also allow a new generation an opportunity to prepare themselves as they *"increase enough"* to possess the land.

During their 40-year circle around the desert, they probably had a few moments when they thought, *"How in the world did we end up here?"* Sometimes it seemed as though I was wandering around in a circle, too, destined to repeat the past and I began to ask myself the same question, *"How did I end up here in the first place?"*

The story of the Israelites departure from their homeland and their decision to go down to Egypt is recorded in the book of *Genesis.* This verse in *Chapter 46:3-4* gives us some important details. *"I am God, the God of your father, He said. Do not be afraid to go down to Egypt, for I will make you into a great nation there. I will go down to Egypt with you, and I will surely bring you back again..."*

When the family first left their home, there was a reason for their departure, a purpose to the journey, and a plan for their return home. The journey out of Egypt and into the Promised Land was just that—a journey home. Egypt was not their home, and neither was the desert. Generations before, their forefather, Jacob (or Israel), and his family had lived in the land of Canaan, but they chose to leave because there was a severe famine in the land. So, they left their homeland and moved to Egypt in search of food.

God used their time in Egypt to grow them into a great nation. But eventually what was meant to strengthen and preserve them began to enslave them. They were going back to their homeland as a changed people. They were no longer who they were before they left Canaan, they were no longer the slaves in Egypt, and they could not enter the Promised Land hanging on to the past. They had some lessons to learn from their past, but they couldn't dwell there.

And so it is with us. The lessons we have learned, can serve to propel us forward into our future. In taking a look at what brought us here, we must also learn how to let go of what is behind and not allow it to rule us. We must remember our past, but we can't dwell there.

In ancient times, famine was considered among one of the worst situations that one could experience. Famines lead people to take drastic measures. Such is the case with the story of the Israelites. They sought an answer to their physical hunger by going in search of food in the land of Egypt. In fact, there are quite a few stories in the bible about people leaving one country and traveling to another in search of food.

I could also add my name to the list of stories about people searching for answers to their hungers. I began to realize I had a few famines of my own. But I discovered that my famines had very little to do with physical hunger. These famines had moved me into a foreign land that seemed to take things from me more eagerly than the promises they made to fulfill.

Ditch the Diets

After years of yo-yo dieting, one of the things I had to examine was the way I thought about food. Our diet and our mindset about food play important roles in finding our proper perception of the role food plays in our lives.

Although our diet certainly does change after surgery, weight loss surgery is not about dieting. It's a lifestyle. The changes we need to make go further than what we're *eating*—it also involves what we're *thinking*.

So, what are we thinking when it comes to food?

What thoughts come to mind when you hear the word "diet"? Dread, anxiety, disappointment, no more fun, pleasure, comfort, or excitement? Will you have to avoid social activities and holiday functions? Will you feel depressed, guilty, or shameful when you do sample rich and tasty fare?

If making changes in our diet for the long-term brings up any feeling of upheaval, throws us into emotional panic, or threatens to leave us a pit of depression, it might be a slight indication that we might be a little off center and that our mindset towards food is off kilter. We need to get our mindset about food and our diet back into balance.

To help visualize this concept, I will use the example of a teeter-totter. Have you ever been sitting on one end of a seesaw with someone sitting on the other end and the other person suddenly gets off? You probably ended up—down on the ground. You were level and balanced as long as there was equal weight on both sides of the bar. Bringing our diet mentality back into balance is like balancing a teeter-totter.

The teeter-totter works on a simple principle. It consists of two parts: a leverage bar and a pivot point. In order for the teeter-totter to be balanced, both of these two elements must be in the proper position.

First, let's take a look at the leverage bar.

In order for the bar to be level it must have equal weight on each side. So, the weight on each side of our leverage bar will represent our former "diet."

The word "diet" has been so misused and misinterpreted in our world. Rather than focusing on balance, we swing from one end of the pendulum to the other: we go "on" a diet, then "off" the diet. Diets have come to mean deprivation to the extreme. We view dieting as a temporary measure until we quickly lose the weight we want so we can resume the way we used to eat. We view food as the enemy and the direct cause of all our problems. We have even adopted the terms "bad" and "illegal" to describe certain food items, and we totally eliminate entire food groups. We think if we eliminate food, we will solve the issue. But it only creates a new one. This dieting extreme is not maintainable. We feel so deprived that all kinds of emotional triggers start to fire. So we "cheat"—ending in over-indulgence, guilt, and self-condemnation. Not to mention the fact that we have labeled ourselves as "cheaters." In an effort to correct our wrong, we repeat the process—again and again.

Our former diets have consisted of huge up and down swings from total deprivation to over indulgence. Like the weights on the teeter-totter, deprivation on one end and over indulgence on the other doesn't equal balance.

Whatever are we thinking?

We need a new food vocabulary, a viewpoint overhaul, and a diet mentality makeover.

After surgery our diet will undergo dramatic changes, but it's not all about limitation.

Even though the quantity of food we can eat will change, the word "diet" in its proper context is defined as a particular selection of food we choose to eat and should be preceded by the word "balanced."

Life from this point on will not be just a plate full of raw green and tasteless lettuce. Nope, salads will not be the staple of your meals. For me, this was good news. We will not have to "diet" anymore. But we will have a new diet. A balanced diet is about *quality* and *selection*. After surgery, the food we *choose to eat* should be based on our goal to be healthy. Our choices should be thoughtfully selected with *occasional* splurges, using wisdom and moderation.

But don't be too hard on yourself, creating a new balance will take time and practice as the *"all or nothing"* mentality is replaced and a new approach to "normal" is recovered.

The Big Pig Out

One day, as I sat at a traffic light, over to my right I could see (out of the corner of my eye) a restaurant that served pork ribs. Not just the small baby backs, but the really BIG ones. The sign reads, *"All you can eat"* and it was calling my name. Pork ribs aren't usually on my routine menu, I do eat them on occasion. But, seriously? All you can eat? What makes me think that *"all you can eat"* is still a good idea? That would only be about two ribs—and small ones at that.

The very idea of unlimited food—why in the world would that idea still exist in my head? It's the same idea as an all-you-can-eat-buffet, only at this particular restaurant you don't even get the exercise benefit of walking to the food. They just bring it to you. What am I thinking?

It's not about the ribs, it's more about an unbalanced mentality— or the, *"all or nothing,"* mentality. I had to rethink the "come to the buffet, eat as much as you want, unlimited food offering."

If my objective is to be successful for the long-term, it means taking a look at how I approach food and bring my thinking back into balance. Just like the teeter-totter, it's much easier to get on and stay on when the leverage bar is in a level position. So, what does that look like exactly?

In a research journal, *Obesity*, a study was done on behavior and psychology by observing people at a Chinese all-you-can-eat-buffet. Findings were made based on the buffet visitor's BMI.

Their observations revealed that people with a higher BMI used larger plates instead of the smaller option. As they approached the buffet, they served themselves before considering all the choices available on the buffet. Not being satisfied with their first hastily chosen selections, they had to make another trip to the buffet. They also observed that those who took a seat facing the buffet, where they could see more food, ate more food. Ninety-four percent of the heaviest people ate all the food they put on their plates. Those who ate with forks instead of chopsticks ate and chewed 11 times faster.

On the other hand, the leaner folks typically made a lap around the buffet first, and considering their choices carefully, they didn't make as many trips. Not only did the thinner folks leave food on their plates, but they ate slower and chewed their food longer.

My observation is that the two groups of people have a whole different approach to the buffet and to their food selection.

Old habits are established from old mindsets. I found that in order to make permanent changes, I needed to look deeper, examining my motives behind *why* I felt attracted to the all-you-can-eat buffet sign in the first place and why I was tempted to overeat.

Q Is the "all-you-can-eat" idea just a habit?

Q Do I feel that I might not get another opportunity to eat?

Q Am I looking for inward satisfaction, with the expectation that food will fill the need?

Q Is it a sense of self-entitlement or rebellion?

Q Is it because I'm an adult, and that I feel it's my right to make my own decisions, unhindered?

Q I do love the taste of food, but why am I not able to control my urge to over-indulge?

Whatever the reason, it gave me a chance to stop and reflect. The ribs are not the problem; it's the deeper issue. I can still eat pork ribs, within limits. I must seek to uncover the root cause of why I think that the sign that states, *"all-you-can-eat,"* still applies to me.

Instead of putting the brakes on food altogether and ending up in deprivation or going full steam ahead into over-indulgence without limits, I found it advantageous to slow down and approach with caution.

It took me a while to realize that my mindset toward food was out of balance. But that was just the first step. I also needed to take a look at what a normal and balanced diet really looks like and be willing to make permanent adjustments.

Q   Am I willing to admit I have an
        unbalanced approach to food?

Q   Do I want to continue living with an unbalanced mindset?

Q   What is normal?

Q   What will normal look like in my everyday life?

Q   How can I start to return food to its proper place?

Q   Am I willing to change my mindset?

Q   How do I change the diet mindset and
        return to normal eating patterns?

Those are very good questions. I'm so glad you asked, because that is just where we're headed!

What Is Normal?

After weight loss surgery, my goal was to return to a normal diet, but I didn't know what *normal* was or how to get there.

Normal? What is "normal" anyway?

I remember this word being used once in a conversation I had with my surgeon, prior to surgery, when I was asking questions regarding gastric bypass surgery. *"Will I be able to eat like a normal person? I just want to be normal."* I suppose the answer I received was, *"Yes."* Thing is, I had no idea what "normal" was.

Here are the synonyms of normal: ordinary, common, customary, being approximately average or within certain limits, a standard. Today's portion sizes may be common and customary, but they have strayed far from card size standard servings that are within the limits of moderation. When it came to my personal portion size, I had strayed far from the norm by making unhealthy adjustments.

Before surgery, I knew a lot about dieting, but that is just the point. Weight loss surgery is not about being on a "diet." After years of "yo-yo" dieting, I had strayed so far from normal that my idea of "normal" was far from accurate.

I didn't realize I was out of balance. Before surgery, even though

> After weight loss surgery, my goal was to return to a normal diet, but I didn't know what *normal* was or how to get there.

diets weren't solving my problems, it was the only plan I knew. My mindset toward dieting led me to believe that my imbalance was perfectly normal. I had to reset my mindset.

In all fairness to "diets," some of those I tried were centered on healthy eating, but the problem was that I didn't make healthy lifestyle changes for the long-term. I was so focused on the foods I couldn't eat, that I totally missed the objective. It was the years of on-again off-again extremes of deprivation and over indulgence that caused problems.

Normal is a relative term. Which means, we only understand normal as it is compared to a particular standard. For example, before surgery, it was normal for me to eat a large bucket of popcorn at a movie. After surgery, I had to establish a new normal, which consists of a few cups. It is very easy to stretch my normal by adding a little more each time. Let's say that I add a cup of popcorn to the amount I eat each time I go to the movie. Each additional cup takes me further and further away from my original starting point. I assess my present position only in comparison to the last increase, not from the original 2-cup starting point and I don't realize how far I've strayed off course. Little by little, my perception of "normal" increases and before long, I'm right back where I started, and eating a large bucket of popcorn seems normal.

Lifestyle and environment play a huge role in establishing our norm. Relatively speaking, a normal and healthy diet for a professional football player is not the same as a normal and healthy diet for an airplane pilot. A healthy diet for a young child is not the same as one for an elderly person. We each have different needs. Our new normal must constitute healthy *bariatric* choices and fit within the guidelines for our newly altered anatomy.

Lifestyle changes will require more than just a change in *what* we eat. After surgery, my *perception of normal* had to change along with my anatomy. My old way of eating may have been my normal, but, I soon learned, I couldn't go back to the old way of eating. Especially here, in the maintenance phase, I couldn't "go back" to that old way of *eating* or my old way of *thinking*." Instead, of wanting

> Weight loss surgery is not about being on a "diet."

to be "normal," or even my idea of "normal," returning to "*balance*" would have been a more accurate objective. Since my goal was to assume a healthy balanced mindset, it was important for me to discover a new bariatric view of "normal."

By the way, even our "normal" bariatric diet changes as we make our way through the process from healing after surgery, weight loss, and then into long-term maintenance. It will require us to make changes in the way we view food and in what is sustainable for us for the long-term.

As these new "normals" are practiced they will form new habits and our new habits will become our new normal way of life.

Balancing Our Diet Mentality

After surgery, I had to change the type of food I was eating, and the amount of food I was eating, but I also had to examine the way I had trained myself to think about food. Not only was my diet out of balance between extreme overindulgence and deprivation, my mindset towards food in general was also off-center. Influenced by years of "yo-yo" dieting I certainly needed a new approach.

This brings us to the second element of the teeter-totter, the pivot point. Just as the leverage bar must be equally balanced, the leverage bar must also be equally spaced and centered on the pivot point. The pivot point is the most important part of the teeter-totter. It's the foundation on which the leverage bar rests.

We will use this pivot point to represent our *diet mentality* or the way we view food as a whole. Just as the pivot point gives the bar stability, accuracy, and support, our mindset must be brought back into alignment so that we too can be stable and strong.

Weight loss surgery allowed me an opportunity to get my diet back to one of moderation, but it also allowed me the opportunity to examine my beliefs about food, which was an important part of the process.

I must admit, I have complained (along with the multitudes) about how incredibly unfair it is that we are doomed to giving up foods which cause us such pain, and, at the same time, comfort. It's better to find out how to redirect our thinking than to be blaming it on the fact that we face eating every day. That fact will not change. What has to change is how we view food and how we use it.

Food is Good

Someone once said that food is an important part of a balanced diet. I agree. Food is not the enemy. Throwing out whole food groups from our diet is like throwing out the baby with the bath water.

We may find that we have made choices based on our perceptions about food or our lack of knowledge based on truth. In our society we are inundated with information, but information changes.

For example, we have been told that butter is bad for us and that we should eat margarine instead. Then we are informed margarine is bad and butter is good. We are warned that eggs raise our cholesterol. Further research reveals eggs are good—if we eat the white and not the yellow. Then we're told, the yellow is good. To our ancestors, bread was the staff of life, but today wheat has become our worst enemy. Everyday there is a new craze, and tomorrow the news may change. We are told that we are fat because we eat too much fat. But, even in the midst of all of the low fat, and low carb deprivation, we have become a more over-weight and under-nourished society. Naturally harvested foods are being replaced by man-made options and we have bought into it. As we continue to stray from the ancient farming practices and soil preservation and continue to drift toward more genetically modified foods, we may continue to find many more food culprits. Until changes are made at the core of the issues, we *must* strive to change our own core beliefs. We must seek the truth about food, considering the healthy benefits that real, whole food is intended to offer us. In addition to that, we need to make wise choices that meet our individual needs, so we can enjoy partaking of it in moderation.

We know that vegetables offer our body nutrition for health. So, what *if* we could eat a vegetable that, when eaten in moderation, offers us more nutrition than calories. What *if* this vegetable was high in fiber, slowed down digestion, contained no fat, kept us fuller longer, and as an added bonus, helped keep us regular. What *if* the phytochemicals in this vegetable helped to lower our cholesterol levels, helped normalize our blood pressure, helped keep our heart healthy, and protected us from disease and oxidative damage. What *if* this same vegetable contained high amounts of vitamins and minerals such as vitamin C, B6, potassium, iron, copper, manganese, magnesium, phosphorus, and folate. And, what *if* this vegetable offered us all that and protein, too. Would we choose to eat it?

Suppose I told you that the vegetable I just described is a white potato. Do you need a minute to reconsider your answer? Although white potatoes have a higher glycemic index, the truth is that potatoes are vegetables. Whole, naturally grown, white foods make up for their pale color by offering abundant nutrition and flavor. When we prepare potatoes boiled, roasted, or baked instead of fried, keep our servings within our new bariatric portion guidelines, choose healthy toppings in moderation, and eat the skin, white potatoes offer us a low-calorie, nutrient and fiber-rich food.

Our case then becomes one of viewing food for its intended purpose. The truth is that food in its original and natural form is one of God's most marvelous creations. It was created to be good for us and pleasurable to us. We were fashioned to enjoy it in all its vast array of tastes, textures, colors, and aromas. It was given to us by God as a lavish gift for our benefit, service, satisfaction, and fulfillment for our physical body—supplying exactly what we need for wellness, growth, and strength. Food is not bad. It is what we have done with it.

In his book, *Soul Survivor*, author Philip Yancey expresses this same idea. He reflects that it may have been one of evil's greatest triumphs to portray the good and enjoyable gifts, which were created and given to us by God, to be bad and God to be the enemy of pleasure.

Food is good. Somewhere along the way, however, we have called upon it to serve us in ways it was never intended. When we abuse it and use it carelessly, even that which was intended to be good possesses the potential to destroy us. Indeed, that which ceases to serve us enslaves us.

My aspiration has become to return to that which is good and to have a balanced view of food and all it offers: life, health, satisfaction, delight, and pleasure.

I encourage you to take some time to think about how you view food and how you feel about making changes for a lifetime. I invite you to educate yourself about nutrition and the requirements of physical health. Take time to reflect on what you believe to be true about food and what it offers you—not based on your *perception* of the *past.*

With a healthy mindset, we can enjoy God's grace and goodness and enjoy the food that was meant to sustain us in our physical body and offer us tremendous enjoyment and pleasure, even after weight loss surgery. No, *Especially* after weight loss surgery.

Changing my mindset about food, eating smaller portions, and choosing healthier options were necessary ingredients of weight loss and maintenance, but, even this didn't solve the entire problem. I couldn't enjoy food and experience inner peace when I was constantly fighting against my desire to eat.

The next step was to discover *why* I was still hungry.

> ... that which ceases to serve us enslaves us.

I'm Still Hungry

I had just celebrated my third year anniversary from surgery. I was learning to adopt a new view of food and my motivation to maintain the weight loss and gain health was strong, but I also faced another challenge. I recognized that the key to my success lay in my ability to make these necessary lifestyle changes, but I began to be aware of my returning appetite and I was finding it hard to remain compliant.

We will all agree that controlling hunger is a major key to compliance. It is much easier to exercise compliance when we are free to choose to make wise food choices. In order to do this, we need to control our appetite.

I know, you thought surgery took care of the appetite issue. Even though weight loss surgery curbs our appetite temporarily, eventually it will return. In order to maintain our accomplishments, it will require us to gain control. So that brings us to the million-dollar question. Actually, there are two questions. *How do we bring our appetite under control? And, if weight loss surgery isn't the answer, then what is?*

In order to answer these questions, it will require that we understand appetites and why we have them. And I do mean *appetites*, plural. We don't have just one appetite. I discovered that we have more than one and it doesn't have anything to do with food. However, if we're struggling with obesity, it could have *everything* to do with food.

I began reading a book by Steven Arterburn and Dr. Debra Cherry, *Feeding Your Appetites: Taking Control of What's Controlling You!* It helped me to understand the many aspects of our appetites.

Some of our desire to eat can be caused by old habits or mindless eating. But most of us recognize that there are other factors that drive us to eat. We are made with an appetite for food, this we know. Although we do need to be compliant to a new way of eating, it's not only about *what* we eat. We must discover *why* we eat.

Of course, we eat when we are physically hungry, but we are not just a physical person. Physical hunger is not the only reason *why* we eat, and physical issues alone are not the sole answer to all our problems. It goes much deeper. We also have an appetite for authority, power, pleasure, work, wisdom, companionship, human interaction, sexual intimacy, love, and acceptance. We also have a desire to be wanted, needed, understood, cared for, appreciated, trusted, and to be in fellowship with God. Wow! No wonder we are still hungry.

We can see that physical hunger is only one part of our makeup. We also have emotional and spiritual hungers.

I believe our appetites are God-given. Not only are we created with several different appetites, but these appetites have value and purpose. I know what you're thinking, *"What purpose could it possibly serve to have all these appetites?"*

Our appetites are beneficial and they fulfill their intended purpose by keeping us healthy in every aspect of our lives. Appetites allow us to live our lives to the fullest—meeting our needs physically, mentally, emotionally, and spiritually.

Our physical appetite helps us get proper nutrition and take pleasure in what we eat. In addition, our mental and emotional appetites stimulate our need for adventure, discovery, exploration, wisdom, peace, companionship, and enjoyment of the world in which we live. Our various appetites allow us to experience emotional, relational, and sexual fulfillment—intimacy, pleasure, and love. They allow us to become fruitful—making sure that the world will go on. In our longing for connection, we can also seek a meaningful relationship with God, which allows us to satisfy our desire for spiritual fulfillment. This ensures that we feel accepted, secure, loved, and significant. Our appetites help to fulfill our needs as a whole person, not just our physical needs.

These appetites were created for our good—that is, when they are in balance. But when they get out of balance, it brings disaster.

As we can see, the appetites that drive us are not just physical and they require more than just physical solutions. Each one of our appetites has a need to be filled. This is where we get off track. We begin to substitute physical solutions, or food in our case, to fill many of our other appetite desires. However, non-physical hungers cannot be satisfied by physical means (or with food). In order to satisfy an appetite, you must use the actual thing that each appetite requires. Our emotional and spiritual hungers will need solutions beyond adjustments in our diet or the alterations of a smaller stomach.

Feeding our other appetites with physical food, leaves them starved, hungry, and ignored. You may have discovered already that our appetites don't like to be ignored. This is when they begin to rage out of control. When left unfulfilled, they can wreak havoc with our ability to reach emotional satisfaction, not to mention long-standing weight loss success.

We must learn to identify our various hungers and fill each one with what they are really longing for. But first, it will be advantageous to learn the difference between real physical hunger and our emotional hungers.

Who's Leading This Caravan, Anyway?

We have spent so much time thinking we're hungry we may not know what true physical hunger feels like.

Physical hunger pangs come from the physical body or stomach. Physical hunger tells us our body is in need of energy or fuel for proper function. We don't go from full to empty all at once. Physical hunger builds gradually and is felt as a growling or burning in the stomach. This hunger is not accompanied by a sense of compulsion or urgency. These hunger pangs will occur several hours after we have eaten a meal. We may start to become aware that we are physically running out of energy. The longer time between meals or the more physically active we are, may be indicators that we may need to eat. Physical hunger softly dissipates when we have eaten and leads to feelings of satisfaction and contentment.

Emotional hunger (sometimes referred to as head hungers) get our attention with loud, overpowering, and sudden screaming in our heads to eat. Emotional hunger strikes suddenly and hits in the mind. It is often triggered by our thoughts, emotions, sight, or smell. It results in an urgent impulse to eat a particular food and is insensitive to time or level of fullness from our last meal. Emotional hunger is distractive with its demands to be heard and after we eat it results in shame and guilt.

I will add, at this point, that the exception to a sense of immediate compulsion or urgency to eat would be a drastic drop in our blood sugar level (or low blood sugar known as hypoglycemia) and will be accompanied by other *physical* symptoms. Continual hunger or feelings of not being satisfied after eating could be an indication of nutritional deficits.

What Is Eating Me?

Once I began to understand my body's different appetites, I began to recognize *why* I wanted to eat.

The first step was identifying the reason why I was looking for food. Was it due to mindless eating habits, true physical hunger, or an unfulfilled emotional need?

- Q Why am I, at this moment, standing in the pantry or looking for food?
- Q At this moment, am I physically hungry?

I discovered that often I was being held captive by emotional eating. I had made substitutions trying to fill my emotional and spiritual hungers with physical food. I needed to change my behavior.

- Q Is eating the choice I really want to make?
- Q Is this what I really want to do?
- Q Will I allow this moment to define my potential or undermine my success?

Making behavioral changes are important, but I had to go a step further than just making outward changes. I had to be willing to determine what brought me to this point in my life in the first place. It meant taking an honest look at the role food played in my life. I had to discover what was at the root of the issues. I had to take a look at the reason *why* I continued to find myself in the pantry looking for food when I wasn't physically hungry. Once again, it's not just about, *"what I'm eating,"* it's more about, *"What is eating me."*

So, how do we discover the root of the problem?

When I find myself standing in the pantry, it is usually because I'm looking for something to sooth life's stresses. Life's stresses,

> Making behavioral changes are important, but I had to go a step further than just making outward changes.

circumstances, and pressures usually trigger emotional eating. The reasons why we react are almost never the present circumstances. Our present circumstances are just the *trigger*. They tend to set off a chain reaction of feelings. Our feelings trigger us to act. Our outward actions are a response to underlying thoughts or core beliefs.

Our actions result in unwanted behaviors. So, how do we eliminate unwanted behaviors?

Famine In the Land

We change our outward by changing our inward. The answers I needed involved uncovering the internal motivations that were behind my actions. I had to discover what was motivating me to eat. If the urge to eat was not physical, it must be coming from my emotions. I had to make the decision to stop and ask myself questions that would help me discover what brought me here.

Q   How am I feeling at this moment?
Q   What am I believing about my circumstances?
Q   What am I believing about myself?

Remember, past beliefs have been laid in a former era. Past hurts that are never allowed to heal hold painful places in our present.

We must be willing to uncover our buried emotions. Dr. Leaf says it this way, *"You can bury your emotions, but you need to know that you are burying something that remains alive."* These buried emotions cannot be controlled, but instead, they control us. Uncovering buried emotions is not always easy and professional help may be required. We must understand that the painful memories of the past, do not hold the ability to hurt us any more than they already have, and ridding ourselves of them will only bring healing and allow us freedom. Believing that they would be better left uncovered, is nothing short of a lie.

Q   When have I experienced feelings like this before?

Next, I had to find the root cause of why I believed what I believed.

Q   Where did this belief originate?

When I determine my core belief, I can examine it in the light of the present truth. This allows me to uproot and pull down false beliefs or past truths that are no longer relevant.

Q   Is the belief true or false?

Q   Is it a past truth, no longer relevant?

Q   Does this thought line up with what I choose to believe about my circumstances?

Q   Does this thought line up with what I choose to believe about myself?

Q   Does this thought line up with what God says about me or my circumstances?

Q   Who's truth will I believe?

Learning to distinguish between physical and emotional hunger and taking the time to ask myself these questions helped me to find the root of what was sending me to the pantry in search for food.

Turning my focus toward issues of inward hunger, I began to discover why I was repeatedly tempted to stray from compliance.

Just as our physical hunger is caused by lack of food, our emotional hungers are caused by a lack of emotional fulfillment. In other words, our unwanted behaviors are most often caused by emotional deficits. We, too, have a famine in our land.

Q   What emotional need do I have at this moment that I am trying to fill with food?

Q   What do I need at this moment to be emotionally satisfied?

Q   What am I really hungry for?

Sometimes we can discover what is at the root of our emotional

> Just as our physical hunger is caused by lack of food, our emotional hungers are caused by a lack of emotional fulfillment.

needs and we can begin to fill our emotional hungers with what they are really in search of.

When we discover the truth about why we are emotionally hungry, we can begin to find a way of escape.

Discovering core beliefs is similar to peeling an onion—you get to the center by removing one layer at a time. As we continue through life we may discover more layers that need to be removed. It is a process that takes time. We can often find solutions to these emotional issues by ourselves, but sometimes the root can be buried deep, well hidden under many years of emotional famines and offences. If so, seeking help from those who are professional experienced in this area will be needed.

When we discover the truth, we can begin to return food to its proper place. When we discover what emotional famines have brought us here, then we can find freedom and we will be free to make the right choices.

Q   What can I do right now, in this moment?
Q   What is the right choice for me?

It is important to remember our past. It can hold some very valuable lessons, but we can't dwell there. We must learn to let go of the past and walk forward into our future.

Just like the example of the teeter-totter, these mindset changes give us leverage. This leverage puts us in the right position and gives us the power and ability to act and to accomplish our task—to maintain the compliance we need to be successful. By constantly monitoring *why* I am motivated to eat, I am able to be compliant to my new way of eating. I am able to maintain proper bariatric portion sizes and focus on nutrition.

I can tell you from experience, that this process is not always easy, but I have found that it is a very important and necessary part of returning to emotional health. Without seeking to determine what brought us here, the end result will be a fleeting moment that doesn't last.

What old labels do I need to lay aside?

....
....
....
....
....
....
....

New positive self-talk

....
....
....
....
....
....
....

What old mindsets do I need to exchange?

....
....
....
....
....
....
....

New truths to embrace

....
....
....
....
....
....
....

".... let us strip off and throw aside every encumbrance (unnecessary weight) and that sin which so readily (deftly and cleverly) clings to and entangles us, and let us run with patient endurance and steady and active persistence the appointed course of the race that is set before us..."

Hebrews 12:1 (AMP)

CHAPTER 30

IX. Thou Shalt Align Thy Expectations and Thy Relationships According to Thy New Likeness

There is a fine line between dreams and reality, it's up to you to draw it.

B. Quilliam

Life for the Israelites wasn't exactly what they expected. They weren't expecting a 40-year detour; they thought they would be in the land of milk and honey by this time, living the "good life," free from battles and hardships. Upon arrival at the border of the land, they thought it would be easy and they would go in and live there, but their relationship with self, others, and their environment had to be adjusted before they could enter the Promised Land. The same is true for us.

For us, the prospect of losing weight and being thin and healthy for a lifetime is exciting, as it should be. But sometimes it may not be all that we imagine. Our satisfaction with weight loss surgery is based on what we are expecting the result to be for the long-term.

I think it is safe to say that we have not had ample experience in maintaining our weight, and considering that weight loss surgery is a whole new experience altogether, it will be important to examine our expectation of what maintenance entails.

Our expectations about what surgery offers us long-term, our relationships with those around us, and our environment can have an undeniable impact on our ability to maintain our weight loss. It will be to our benefit to take a look at our expectation of what we *think* weight loss surgery offers us and consider the whole experience in its proper perspective.

Our satisfaction with weight loss surgery is based on what we are expecting the result to be for the long-term.

Q   What do you anticipate that your long-term results will look like?

Q   Do you think you will lose all of the weight and keep it off—forever?

Q   Do you believe that keeping the weight off will be easy?

Q   Are you expecting the surgery to do all the work?

Q   Do you believe that you will be free from temptations?

Q   Do you expect all your dependencies to just disappear?

Q   Do you anticipate that you will be healthy and not experience health problems again?

Q   Are you ready for the weight loss phase to end?

Q   Will you face weight regain?

Q   Do you know what long-term maintenance will require?

Q   Are you willing to accept the realistic expectation of what weight loss surgery really entails?

Q   Are you ready and willing to accept the responsibility of maintenance?

You might be surprised that your answers to these questions may not be a true representation of what life is like after surgery. After working so hard to reach my weight loss goals, I expected to be healthy and remain healthy once and for all. I thought that after reaching my lowest weight that I would keep it off and never have to face weight regain—but I was wrong.

"We're NOT in the Promised Land. Yet. But we will get there. First, however, our idea of what surgery offers us may need a little expectation adjustment.

Yes, We Do

Weight loss brings change to all areas of our lives and our relationships are no exception. There will be changes and challenges to both casual relationships as well as to those who are the closest to us—and especially so in marriage. In the book, *Weight Loss Surgery for Dummies*, it is reported that, *"Weight loss surgery makes good marriages better and bad marriages worse. Unfortunately, the incidence of divorce among weight loss surgery patients is higher than the average."*

We often hide behind weight as an excuse for why our relationships aren't working. Once the weight is gone we may discover the weight was not the problem. It will be helpful to re-examine our goals and desires for our relationships and approach them with realistic expectations.

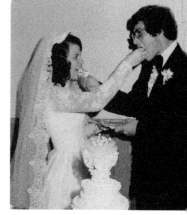

1975

Q   Do you imagine that losing weight will cure all of your relationship issues?

Q   Do you believe those around you will be as thrilled with your weight loss success as you are?

Q   Will people continue to compliment you and recognize your success?

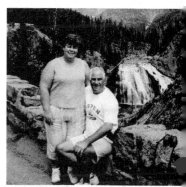

2004

Q   Do you expect that you will be changed by your weight loss?

Q   Do you expect that others will be changed by your weight loss?

Q   Do you think that all your friends will be happy for you?

Q   Can you imagine that some of your friends might even be jealous of your success?

Q   Do you think that your spouse will talk to you more, initiate intimacy more often, or become more romantic as a result of your weight loss?

Q   Do you think that your entire family will approve of the new you?

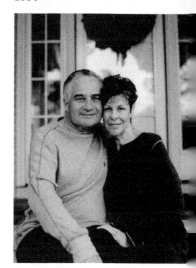

2007

> # Food doesn't fulfill all our needs. Weight loss won't fulfill all our needs, and neither do relationships fulfill all our needs.

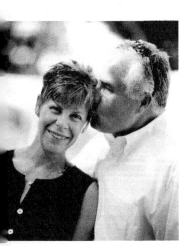

June 2008

While in the weight loss phase, you will receive lots of compliments and attention. Everything is new and exciting. But in long-term maintenance, the "new you" will soon become the "old you". The compliments wane because people are used to seeing you as you are in the present. My children (who were adults when I had weight loss surgery) relate that they no longer remember me being overweight. My friends no longer remark on how great I look. Some of them encourage me to gain weight because I am "too thin". In fact, friendships that were established after I had lost weight never knew the "old me." They didn't see me when I weighed over 300 pounds and they don't value my accomplishments with the same enthusiasm as the ones who knew me before I lost weight.

There is a great possibility that your relationships could change drastically or, perhaps disappointingly, remain the same or worsen. If we are looking to weight loss to eliminate relational difficulties that existed beforehand, we might want to look again. In the same manner, if we are expecting relationships to satisfy all our needs or fulfill our emotional deficits, we will also need to reconsider. Food doesn't fulfill all our needs. Weight loss won't fulfill all our needs, and neither do relationships fulfill all our needs. Weight loss itself is rarely the answer to relationship issues. Just as with our weight loss commitments, both casual and intimate relationships require intentional and purposeful diligence for success.

My husband and I have been married for more than 38 years, and like all couples we experience ups and downs in our relationship. My husband expected that all our problems would disappear after I lost weight and that our marriage would be perfect. It's not. Even though he is extremely proud of my accomplishments, an indispensible supporter, and my greatest encourager, our challenges were not all weight related and we still have some of the same challenges we had before I lost weight. However, our marriage has gotten stronger since my weight loss surgery, but it has very little to do with my weight loss. Our marriage improved as a result of a mutual decision to be diligent, attentive, and committed to each other. Marriage is more than a physical, weight-based relationship or an emotional connection—marriage is a spiritual bond. Both extra weight and weight loss can magnify the good and the bad in a marriage, but it is up to you and your spouse to decide if you are willing to work on your relationship as you both change over time.

Environmental Challenges

Have you noticed how things in our environment such as the weather or music affect the way we feel? The environment around us really does rub off on us. It can promote positive emotions or trigger negative ones.

To live successfully in the new land will require us to make a few environmental modifications. I found that I had to lay aside everything that wasn't absolutely necessary to operate successfully in my new lifestyle. But let's face it. When we arrive at the long-term maintenance phase, we will continue to live in the real world. There are temptations all around us. We can't always control, change, or avoid everything in our environment, but there are things we *can do*.

Setting ourselves on a course for success will require a little "house cleaning." I don't just mean cleaning out the cupboards and the refrigerator. We often need to examine other influences in our surroundings. This involves clearing away old dependencies, limiting time in dangerous surroundings, and freeing ourselves from negative influences. It may be time to consider if there is anything in our *environment* that is holding us back.

Q Does your environment hold temptations?

Q What things can you eliminate that are unnecessary distractions or temptations for your long-term success?

Q Are you prepared to confront the things in your environment that you can't eliminate?

Q Are you prepared to face birthday parties, Thanksgiving dinners, holiday celebrations, Easter,

Christmas, family get-togethers, movies, baby showers, graduations, funerals, The Forth of July, The Fifth of May, The Sixth of September, backyard cookouts, lunch at the office, the county fair, potlucks, or life in general? How will you handle it?

Q Are you prepared for the temptations that lurk down the grocery store aisles?

Q Will you ever drive by your favorite restaurant, bakery, or ice cream shop again?

Q Are there things from the past that hold negative influences or prompt old behaviors to arise?

Q Will there be places from the past that stir up negative feelings or provoke old behaviors?

Q What will you allow to define you?

Of course, your environment holds temptations. I've said it before, but it bears repeating. All of the relational issues, marital issues, temptations, and triggers we had before surgery were not removed with the rerouting of our gut.

We can make an effort to eliminate the things we can, but there will be a whole world of things we can't change. I have found that when I can't change my circumstances, it becomes necessary to change my response as well as my expectations. It became necessary to prepare myself to face the immovable, give some thought to how I was going to respond to the factors I couldn't change, and discover how to create a safer environment.

The Web of Sabotage

The Israelites found that when they allowed themselves to be swayed by the false beliefs and opinions of others it prevented them from possessing their promise.

It's easy to let others define our boundaries or rule our choices. I also found myself conforming to the subtle expectations of others at times. I discovered that, in some areas, I was allowing someone else to rule me. This is especially true in the early months after surgery. I made the choice to eat when I was stressed, pressured, or when my feelings or weaknesses were getting the best of me.

Q Are there any people from your past that encourage or ignite negative behaviors?

Q Do you think that others might knowingly or unknowingly attempt to sabotage you?

Q Are you prepared for the possibility that the people who remain in your life, namely spouse, parent, children, family, friends, etc. may inadvertently sabotage you?

Q Will you allow others to define you?

It's so easy to get caught in the web of sabotage. Just like spider webs, they seem to show up in places you didn't even know a spider existed. Sometimes they span across spaces that make you wonder how they were even constructed in the first place. They seem to appear out of nowhere, quickly make themselves right at home, build in every available corner, and multiply beyond belief. Or sometimes we find a cobweb—you know, one that has been there for a while, only we never recognized it until it was covered with dust.

The strength of a web is in its design. A spider web is unbelievably strong and durable. They are uniquely constructed to withstand hurricane force winds, and strategically placed and well hidden to catch prey off guard. Sabotage works in a similar way. By definition, sabotage is a deliberate action designed to weaken another, often by applying pressure.

I'm sure you recognize these webs of sabotage. Some have been there all along. Our best friend, spouse, mother, mother-in-law, or even our own self-talk may apply to our pressure points. *"I made it just for you." "Are you going to waste it?" "Just this one time won't hurt." "You've lost enough weight, you look under-nourished." "You're too thin." "You need to eat."* I have found that almost every occasion holds an excuse to get caught in the web of sabotage. As if I need any help. I seem to get into enough trouble on my own—any time, season, or circumstances will do.

Whether intentional or unintentional, peer-driven or self-induced, new or old, these webs are also intricately designed and well disguised. When strategically placed, they appeal to our weakness and can throw us off guard, leaving us vulnerable and entangled in feelings of guilt, shame, or self-condemnation.

> **Q** Do you think you will be exempt
> from sabotaging yourself?
>
> **Q** Are you expecting the surgery alone to do all the work?

Although I make my own choices, early on, it didn't take much to sabotage my best intentions. We need to know how to avoid getting tangled in one of these traps. It only takes a fine mist or a little dust to reveal a spider web and so it is with these webs of sabotage. With a little know how, we can be armed and ready to detect, avoid, or combat them.

Forming new habits is not just about what we *do*, it also involves the way we *think*.

Avoiding the Webs of Sabotage

Instead of conforming to the world around us, I found a better option was to transform or change my environment and my way of thinking. In the pre-surgery phase, we discussed how important it is to have a strategy and construct a plan of action. This will allow us to form new lifestyle habits. Forming new habits is not just about what we *do*, it also involves the way we *think*.

Assess, Decide, and Prepare

Knowing the opposition and where it might exist, allows me to form a plan of action. First, I determine whether I can change the situation or if there are adjustments I *can* make, if any.

Making sure the environment is clear of negative influences sometimes calls for subtle changes or I may find the need to take more drastic measures. Sometimes, I find it necessary to put an end to unwanted ills in my environment by closing the door to temptation altogether. At other times, I can limit my time with those around me who have a history of sabotaging my efforts. But there are situations that can't be avoided. In this case, I must be prepared to make changes in the way I respond.

Q   What *can* I do?

I can control myself, the way I think, and the way I respond. If I don't choose to rule my emotions, my emotions will rule me. I had to learn not to be caught off guard. I had to practice the scenarios ahead and be prepared. *"What will I do if….?"* I find it best not to wait until I am in the heat of the moment to make these decisions. I must have a pre-determined course of action.

I Can Strengthen My Internal Resolve

I must define my internal convictions and motivations. My motivation to change must be stronger than the desire to stay where I am. I must give myself a reason to act. My motives are the driving force behind my actions.

I decide what I want. I start by revisiting my reasons to remain compliant or my overall incentives for having weight loss surgery in the first place. This strengthens my resolve and will serve to keep me determined, focused, armed, and alert.

My long-term objective is to find improved health and achieve a balanced mindset. I must stay focused on the commitment I made to take care of myself and to make healthier lifestyle choices.

Q   What is my objective?
Q   Why did I have surgery?
Q   What is my motivating factor?
Q   Is my motivating factor strong?
Q   What are my long-term objectives?
Q   What do I really want?

> I can control myself, the way I think, and the way I respond. If I don't choose to rule my emotions, my emotions will rule me.

Q Do I have an action plan for how to respond in this situation?

Q What are the convictions that hold me to my plan?

Q Am I motivated by pleasing other people who tempt me to do things outside my boundary or am I motivated by my desire to remain healthy and keep my weight under control?

Q What *can* I do?

When other people around me overstep their boundary, and pressure me with their own expectations, I don't have to allow these situations to cause me to step outside of the boundaries I have established for my success. I have to strengthen my ability not to be easily persuaded.

I've had to find cleaver and creative ways to maneuver through and around these situations—replacing opportunities to give in, with opportunities to be strong. I can't give in to the expectations of others. I ask myself what actions I *can* take to ensure I stay true to my convictions and my objectives.

I Can Know My Limits and Define My Boundaries

In the beginning, there were a lot of things I forbid my husband to bring into the kitchen. If he wanted a candy bar, I requested he eat it elsewhere. As time passes, it doesn't pose the same temptation. I'm no longer tempted to eat candy bars. When we go grocery shopping together, my husband becomes an ice cream magnet, but ice cream doesn't usually tempt me beyond my ability to control.

I am able to take a few bites of cake, and be done. But, when it came to donuts, it took a long time to get to that point. For over six years I had to place a strict boundary around donuts. I couldn't even be in the same room with a donut, or things wouldn't turn out well. I was really glad that the Krispy-Kreme Donut Store location was all the way across town so I was less tempted to make the trip. I actually was very annoyed when I realized that their donuts could be purchased in the grocery store. Then Dunkin' Donuts placed a drive thru location just across the street. As a general rule, Dunkin' Donuts didn't tempt me, but the convenience of the drive-thru certainly did. It meant my territory was being invaded and my resolve was being tested.

Avoiding donuts forever was not an option. Those little bags of powdered sugar varieties pop up without warning at any grocery story aisle intersection. Once I see them, it's all I can do to avoid putting them in my cart. I had to learn to strengthen my fortitude. I had to retrain my mind to shift gears, from donuts to the task at hand. I had to make it a habit to call up my motivating factors immediately and without delay.

I can say that during the last few years, I have tasted a donut once or twice, and I know I have a weakness for them. The decision to taste them is well thought out and strategically planned. It's not based on an irresistible whim. Until I could eat them within the limit, I tried to avoid them like the plague and I learned to redirect my thinking and form a plan of action when I was tempted.

Just because I permit myself a few bites of the occasional dessert, it doesn't mean I always give in. I often face opportunities to indulge. Once I attended a holiday dinner where the hostess had baked a cake, "*just for me.*" Careful thought had been taken to alter the recipe with a certain ingredients in hopes it would be acceptable. But before the event, I had already made up my mind to stay on my plan. Once I arrived, I surveyed my options and made my selection. I looked forward to enjoying the items that were safely within my boundary. Even though the cake was offered with goodhearted intentions, it was neither within my bariatric-friendly guideline nor my personal perimeters. I graciously conveyed my thanks for their thoughtfulness. I enjoyed the beautiful presentation of the dessert and complimented them on how yummy it looked. But being very satisfied with my decision and very determined to stick to my plan, I politely turned down the offer to eat it. There were plenty of other people who did enjoy eating it.

I Can Be Vigilant

I must be willing to do what it takes to be successful. I am constantly confronted with temptations. I must remain constantly aware of potential pitfalls and remain vigilant and focused on the things that are important. I remind myself to take one day at a time.

Over the years, I have learned a few valuable lessons including that contentment is a choice. When my circumstances cannot be changed, I must learn to change my mind.

Easy? Certainly not. It isn't easy. It's not easy now, and living life in the new land long-term will not be easy, either. We will need to be strong and courageous. However, making a few adjustments now will be easier than facing the folly of leaving things to chance in the years ahead. We didn't choose the "easy" road, but this one will place us on the right path to possess our Promised Land and in the end it will reward us the greatest potential to enjoy ongoing success.

CHAPTER 31

X. Thou Shalt Not Be Ruled By Weight Regain, Fear, or Other Masters

Insanity: doing the same thing over and over again and expecting different results.

Albert Einstein

By the end of their four hundred year stay in Egypt, the Israelites had grown stronger in number. But not only had they become slaves under the rule of the Pharaoh, they had also allowed themselves to be controlled by other rulers—fear and non-belief.

I often wonder why the Israelites didn't leave Egypt when things started to go wrong. What kept them there? Had their fear of starvation kept them enslaved in cruel living conditions? Were they so deceived and entangled that they didn't believe there was a way of escape?

Once out of captivity, the Israelites not only allowed themselves to be held captive by their former beliefs, they also sabotaged themselves by conforming to the beliefs of those around them. Before God could lead them into the Promised Land, the Israelites had to be free of all of the things that "ruled" them.

Gaining possession was determined by their ability to eliminate this internal corruption. They had to be willing to overthrow the inhabitants that awaited them in the new land. They needed to be strong and courageous. But instead of courage, the people began to be overtaken by fear. Along with their non-belief, their fear obstructed their entrance into the land. They had to rid themselves of the strongholds of the past and learn to trust in a new way of life. They had to face their fear and be emotionally equipped to confront what lay ahead.

We have taken a look at the things that brought us here, but we must also take a look at what keeps us here. Following the example of the Israelites, in our going forward, we must ask ourselves, *"What is still ruling us?"*

Winning the Battle of Regain

Remember, weight loss surgery is a great tool for helping us get a jumpstart on weight loss, especially for those of us who seem to struggle against all odds of ever being successful. But as glorious as our Promised Land looks from a distance, upon a closer inspection, there are a few things that still stand in the way of our success. One of these is the giant-sided aspect of weight regain.

You have got to be kidding me! Weight gain after gastric bypass? What next? And we thought plateaus were hard.

Will we gain back weight during long-term maintenance? Let's look at the facts.

It is true that our weight may shift as we find our long-term normal. Studies show that 35 to 50 percent of patients who undergo gastric bypass will regain weight. On average, most people will regain approximately 10 percent of their lowest-achieved weight during this normalization process. This is not a declaration that you will gain or a justification to gain weight back, but the possibility is real. Studies also show that after 10 to 14 years, 60 percent of the excess weight loss has been maintained with RNY.

There are numerous dynamics at work that cause reoccurrence of weight. The increase in body weight during this maintenance phase is not completely understood. Weight regain after surgery is based on many factors such as pre-operative body mass index, nutritional habits, self-esteem, mental health, socioeconomic status, fistula formation, increases in portion sizes, as well as non-compliance to diet and exercise. But bariatric surgeons believe that possible internal changes in the anatomy of the stomach and the dilatation of the stoma may also play a role in RNY patients. This occurs when the stomach pouch and the opening to the small intestine (the stoma) stretch over time, allowing one to eat more without feeling full. In other words, weight regain is not always within our control.

We must also take into consideration that we haven't had too much practice at this maintaining thing. It will take time to learn to balance our food intake and our activity level. During the weight loss phase, we have not only lost fat but we have also lost muscle mass. As we continue to build our muscle mass, we may experience a shift in our weight.

And just when you think you have it all figured out, things change. I can tell you from experience that you can expect your body to change for many years. Just as we discussed with plateaus, our body's metabolism plays a key role in our weight. As we grow older our metabolism slows down and we may find it more difficult to maintain our weight.

 Emotional issues can also play a key role in the return of head hunger. It is a great time to examine those inner motivations and triggers to emotional hunger. It may also be a good time to examine your boundaries as well as to become conscious of any old habits that might have crept back in. Unless you are being recklessly non-compliant to the guidelines, a weight increase should *not* be viewed as a *failure* or your *fault*.

Whatever the cause, weight regain is an emotionally disturbing experience to a formerly overweight person. When I started to experience regain after several years, my husband reminded me that I was told about this in the beginning; however, it's quite hard to accept when you're going through it.

Patients (including myself) often see our lowest achieved weight as a benchmark for success. This perception can lead to long-term dissatisfaction and perceived failure. These thoughts lead one to think that things aren't any different than before surgery and that we will once again end up back where we started. The bottom line is that during this phase, some regain is expected; and as we age the possibility of weight regain increases. It will be to our advantage to learn how to accept the possibility of weight regain if, or more likely WHEN, we find ourselves in this dilemma. We must learn to identify any potential untrue thoughts that threaten to sabotage us, and prepare ourselves to defeat them by aligning ourselves with the truth.

Putting weight regain into perspective means viewing our overall understanding of success. When we view regain as a failure we sabotage ourselves. We often say that the surgery doesn't work. The truth is, the surgery does work. It just doesn't work all by itself. It works along with hard work on our part and our facing the responsibility and the commitment that losing weight and maintaining the loss requires.

Now, let's get real. Our stomach was changed to the size of a walnut. And yes, over time, our pouches stretch. We can't condemn ourselves for that, it's part of the healing process. But studies show that pouch size is not a measure of success and neither is regain.

I did accept the fact that I might experience a small weight gain. I didn't expect a tremendous battle with low blood sugar levels. There were a few years that I struggled to balance my eating, exercise, and blood sugar and I started to experience regain. I didn't want to accept the fact that I had regained 20 pounds, but those 20 pounds turned into 30 pounds. It brought with it feelings of frustration, disappointment, and failure. Even though my regain was partly due to my uncontrollable blood sugar levels, it would have been easy for me to throw in the towel and say the surgery didn't work. The surgery did work. It did the job of helping me lose the weight, and I had to be willing to continue do the work of keeping it off. Now that my blood sugar levels are more stable, I must be willing to do as much exercise as my condition will allow. I have to accept the limitations of which I have no control.

I must continually remind myself to put things into perspective. I have been successful. For over seven years after surgery, I kept off more than 130 pounds. I also had to accept the fact that I was 7 years older. I improved my health and I established a new life. When I dwell on the regain and the misfortune of hypoglycemia, I cheat myself out of my successes.

Even though it's easier said than done, we should strive not to let weight gain rule our emotions to the point where we give up, allow ourselves to slide back into non-compliance, affect our self-worth, or determine our success. It is important to put our weight loss experience, improved health, and quality of life into their proper perspective and not let regain or unrealistic expectations rule us.

The Five-Foot Ruler

Some years ago, I discovered a hilarious greeting card. It had a picture on the front of a woman standing on a scale and inside the card read, "*I gotta buy some lighter underwear.*" I bought it for myself. If there is one thing I can identify with, it is the emotional weighing game. It also reminds me of how silly it is to get so bent out of shape when the scale starts to move.

If you have done any research at all regarding how often you should weigh yourself, you'll find everyone has a different opinion. Some believe that weighing too often sets us up for failure. However, studies show that people who weigh everyday are more likely to keep their weight off. Whatever side we are on, we need to put our idea of weighing ourselves back into balance.

We do need to establish boundaries. I have established a boundary for my weight within a 5-to-7 pound range. This accounts for normal fluctuations, but too far in the wrong direction and I know I must evaluate my diet and activity to find out *if* I have strayed off course.

I routinely step on the scale every morning before breakfast. It is a good plan and it really works well, or at least, I thought it did. That was, until the day I realized I was allowing that five-foot piece of metal to rule my emotions.

If my weight was up, I was discouraged, sometimes for days or weeks, until it moved in the downward direction. If I lost, I was pleased.

The scale is not the problem and neither is weighing every day. Although numbers are important in measuring our position, success is not based on numbers and weight loss alone.

I have found that, contrary to popular belief, the scale isn't a fair judge and it doesn't always tell the whole truth. It can give me my weight for the moment, but it changes its mind as often as I change clothes. It changes after I eat breakfast. It changes from morning to night. It changes when I eat too much salt or soy sauce. The scale can't tell me if my weight gain or loss is due to water, fat, or muscle. It doesn't report the state of my health or my mental condition. It only gives the truth in pounds, as it knows it; that much is true. It can reveal the consequences of eating that piece of cake, but it can't tell me *why* I ate it.

The scale is a tool, not a rule. The tool should help me set my boundaries and achieve my goals. The problem becomes when I allow the numbers to rule my emotions. I realized I had the power to choose to rule my emotions and change my thoughts.

During the weight loss phase, I had to accept that fluctuations were a normal part of the process as my body adjusted to the chemical and biological changes that were occurring. I also had to accept that fluctuations, and even regains, were a part of maintenance. There is evidence that suggests that weight loss surgery patients experience more weight fluctuation than normal, especially in the maintenance phase.

I did experience weight regain within several years after reaching my lowest weight.

With that said, as a part of my maintenance program, I still keep a close eye on the scale. I still weigh myself everyday and I still have a boundary range. I continually take into consideration my overall progress and health—taking inventory of my food intake and my activity level. And I continually have to remind myself not to give the scale or the numbers the power to defeat me.

I am constantly aware of and consider the motivation behind how often I weigh and why?

Q Am I motivated by fear or failure?

Q Does weighing or not weighing send me on an emotional roller coaster?

Q Do I have a sense of peace?

Q Does weighing motivate me to do my best or does it drive me into unbalanced behavior?

Q Do I fear the numbers on the scale?

Q What am I afraid of?

We must be careful not to let the numbers rule us. Weigh-ins can be emotional triggers that send us wayward. Along with daily weigh-ins, I feel that it is important to consider my overall objectives and keep things in the proper perspective. I routinely journal my food intake and remember to "keep the main thing the main thing" which is my overall progress and health. I encourage you to do the same.

What is right for someone else may not be right for you. Your level of health should be determined by your surgeon and health care professionals in relation to your overall health, individual medical history, and personal goals—not peer pressure or someone else's unqualified opinion of what is best for you.

This can also apply to other areas of our health. When my cholesterol numbers started to come down my cardiologist was extremely delighted and amazed at my progress. Although my numbers were still a little higher than I thought ideal, he explained that my success in relation to my past medical history, as well as family history, was within the expected, acceptable, and healthy limit.

And so it is with our weight. We must take into account our unique circumstances and bring our expectations into the correct perspective. Our goal after surgery must be based on achieving the best level of health that is within our power to achieve—in every area of our lives. We all must find what is best for us, individually.

> Your level of health should be determined by your surgeon and health care professionals in relation to your overall health, individual medical history, and personal goals— not peer pressure or someone else's unqualified opinion of what is best for you.

Therefore, measuring our success by the numbers on the scale, the size of our stomachs, the size of our clothes, or even lighter underwear, doesn't give us the whole picture. Our mental attitude, how we see ourselves, and the thoughts we think regarding the weight loss experience as a whole are just as vital. These will directly determine our long-term outcome.

Don't Be Ruled By the Rules

Although weight loss surgery comes with its own set of rules and guidelines for health, we may find that we are lugging around a lot of rules that should have been long forgotten. When it comes to food, we need to examine our motivation behind why we do what we do and unload our unending supply of dieting rules.

Not only has our diet mentality told us food was bad, following the rules has become a way of measuring ourselves—making us feel "bad" about who we are.

I was talking with my friend, Lisa, about her experience after weight loss surgery. She didn't realize until after she had surgery that her diet mentality was holding her back from enjoying healthy food. Being caught up in years of diet mentality, she had eliminated all of her choices by having to obey the diet rules. In the process, she was constantly condemning herself. *"Every diet I ever went on had a different set of rules, and I had adopted them all, and the rules were ruling me. I had no freedom of choice other than to obey them because I was being motivated to be 'good' by following them."*

For example, we know that eating endless amounts of dessert is not a wise choice for health, but an occasional bite of desert should not be detrimental to our cause. When we do choose to taste an occasional sweet treat, we don't need to condemn ourselves for our actions, assume feelings of guilt, or punish ourselves with total deprivation. Remember, food is not "bad" and it doesn't make us "bad" when we eat it.

Condemnation pronounces us incurable and continually points out our failure and how badly we've messed up. Condemnation binds us to the problem and makes no separation between us and our actions. All the while, it threatens and accuses us with judgment and disapproval, and leaves us feeling trapped with no solution or way of escape. These inner voices tell us, *"You're no good,"* or, *"You're not worth it, why do you even try,"* or, *"You're a failure."* These allegations leave us feeling discouraged, rejected, and worthless—causing us to live in despair without hope.

Lisa found she was being held captive by the rules. It wasn't until she started asking herself why she was following the rules in the first place that she realized her motivation was out of alignment.

Q   How do I feel about myself when I eat certain foods?
Q   Does eating a certain food make me feel "bad," "guilty," or "shameful?"
Q   Why am I following the rules in the first place?
Q   Do I follow the rules for the sake of the rules or do I follow them because rules are a model for success?

Both Lisa and I have discovered that we had to lay aside our diet mentality or emotional baggage that came with letting the rules rule us.

Change must first come from the inside out. In order to return to balance, our *perception* of the rules has to change and our objective must be to find our true motivating factor.

Just like the Ten Commandments offer us guidelines for success, our bariatric rules offer us guidelines for successful eating. Following the rules is the choice we make based on our personal values and our ultimate goal—to be successful and healthy.

We can start by being willing to educate ourselves about the value of whole food and what it offers us. This knowledge, combined with our desire to pinpoint our overall objective, and our intentional effort to find our motivating factors will allow us to make wise choices and reward us with good health.

With all of this in the proper perspective, we will be provided a sound relationship with food—allowing us to *choose* an occasional variation from the norm, such as a bite or two of dessert, or a few French fries, without being held captive by feelings of shame and guilt. We simply make a choice to move forward and make corrections if and when they become necessary. It will permit us to drop all the oppressive, guilt-ridden, diet-driven vocabulary such as, *"I shouldn't have eaten that..."* or *"I should have done better,"* or *"I was so 'bad' to have eaten that..."*

Embracing the rules as a pathway to living a healthier life will assist us in leaving behind our emotional baggage and move us a few steps closer to freedom from obesity.

Don't Be Ruled By Fear

We have seen that the pre-surgery phase is overloaded with a wide variety of stresses, fears, and uncertainty, but these aren't just limited to pre-surgery. As weight loss surgery patients we may face many fears throughout the process. Dealing with fear is a very real and normal part of recovery after weight loss surgery. I had to face the fears of the past and even fears of the future. Fear of failure, fear of weight regain, fear of exposure, fear of not being good enough, or perfect enough, loved enough, strong enough, disciplined enough, or just simply–not enough.

Most of my fears before surgery were unfounded, but nevertheless these concerns appeared very real and overwhelming when I was going through them.

I faced a fear of eating after surgery. At first, my fear was based on protecting my pouch. I was able to set aside my apprehension after being encouraged by my surgeon that it was safe to leave the clear liquid stage and move to the full liquid stage.

I still have to face feelings of fear. One includes returning to obesity. It is so easy to let fear take over, tempting me to swing from one extreme to another—from overeating to skipping meals or not eating enough.

Fear is one of our greatest enemies. Just as fear robbed the Israelites of a speedy entry into their Promised Land, fear can rob us, too. Fear immobilizes us and keeps us from accomplishing our greatest potential. It steals our joy, our peace, and our security. It deprives us of love, personal identity, and a healthy self-worth. It robs us of our wealth, destroys our health, and even shortens our life.

I once heard an acronym that helped me identify this unwanted fear. FEAR is False Evidence Appearing Real. It's when we allow our thoughts to convince us that something is true, when in reality, it's false. It really doesn't have any power to hold us—it just makes us think it does.

If fear is false evidence appearing real, then indeed it is just an appearance. Fear is an emotion or feeling brought on by a *perceived threat* or something that we *believe* to be true. Most of the time it has very little to do with facts, yet, it can seem real, very, very real. Our *perception* of truth is based on our life experiences and things that might have been true in the past, but they may no longer be the truth for our present.

Fear makes our challenges look larger and more frightening that they really are. It hides the truth and builds its foundation on falsehoods. It deceives us with past truths, trying to persuade us that things in the past are also true in the present. Playing our past experiences over and over in our mind, it convinces us of our failures and tells us we have no options, recourse, or escape.

Time also has a way of distorting the memories of the past. The further we move from the memory, the more likely it is to become out of focus. We still recall the events, but details may be a little less exact and the emotions attached to the memories may grow more intense.

We don't automatically let go of those memories and emotions. As we move on through life the impact of those events carry a great influence in our lives. Those old memories grow weaker, but they appear very strong. These weak recollections are a foundation upon which all of the thoughts, emotions, and circumstances of our present are erected.

Getting to the root of my issues required going back to the beginning to where it all got started. Remember, it's ok to recall the past as long as we don't dwell there.

Q   So what do we fear?

Q   Are our fears real or imagined?

Q   Are they past or present?

My past held old graves of insecurity, which although buried deep, were never really buried at all, but remained fresh and haunted me like recurring nightmares.

My grandfather, Papa Webb, died when I was about 18 months old. I still remember standing at the door awaiting his daily visits. I may have been young, too young actually, to understand the sudden and tremendous loss of love and security, but I certainly felt it.

My mother went back to work soon after. I remember vividly the deep sense of helplessness and hopelessness I felt every time my mother left me. Years later those memories repeatedly tore at my unhealed wounds of insecurity and renewed themselves with separation anxiety as I began attending kindergarten. They remained strong through years of grade school—growing more prevalent during the years my father suffered from the debilitating illness that threatened his life. Every morning when I left for school I wondered if it might be the last time I would see him. My fears were confirmed in January of 1970, when my dad passed away of a sudden and fatal heart attack. I was 12 years old. I was very close to my dad. I was his little shadow. It was a huge traumatic experience for us all. My dad was a very affectionate person, much more so than my mom, so I received most of my physical affection as well as emotional security from my dad. As I watched my mom cope with the tremendous loss, and being the oldest child, I assumed the responsibility for her happiness and I became more and more insecure.

I carried those feeling of insecurity and even abandonment into adulthood, into my marriage, and into the present. They presented themselves with constant triggers and preyed on every available opportunity to be revived—each time bringing with them a host of other fiends just as ominous.

No matter how large or small these old wounds may appear

they grow nevertheless. Some may appear dead, in scantly marked graves, lying dormant and well-hidden while others stand like monuments marking traumatic incidences that are decades old— breaking the ground as they arise with more intense vengeance and overwhelming emotion than when they were first laid.

We all have emotional graveyards in our lives. The battle begins in our thoughts. The war against fear has to be fought and won in our mind. Imagined or real, our body doesn't know the difference. It creates disillusionment and despair, produces stress, and causes us to turn to food. Stress also releases hormones that can wreak havoc in our body and have an adverse affect on our ability to lose weight and keep it off.

There is something to be said for facing our greatest fears. Learning how to deal with emotional turmoil, and the physical effects it can have on our health, can be beneficial to long-term success. We don't just need to know how to cope with our fears, we need to know how to conquer them.

So how do we conquer our fears?

I start by asking myself what I am feeling, especially when I find myself looking for food when I'm not hungry. Then I ask myself when the feeling started. Once I find the answer, I ask myself what I believe about my situation and about myself. Then I asked myself if this belief is a truth or a lie.

Once I recognize what the untruth is, I can start to replace those thoughts with true thoughts. I start by saying to myself, "Yes, it is true that I once failed at weight loss, but today is a new day. Today I can make the choice not be ruled by my past failures. I have the opportunity to make another choice. I will not live in the past. I will live in the now. I cannot undo the past, but I can make a different choice today."

I encourage you to think on things that are true and worthy of your time, thoughts that are excellent and of a good report, thoughts that will put you on the winning side, thoughts that will bring you peace. Give yourself a good shot of encouragement.

What do you believe? Is what you believe true, real and present truth? What do you choose to believe?

Freedom is based on finding truth. Once we find the lie behind our false belief, we can find freedom. It may take time and effort, or even professional help, but we can be free.

For the Israelites, the trip into Egypt was not for their demise. God had a plan to use their time there to make them stronger. And, so it is with us.

Weight loss surgery gives us the tool we need to succeed. It gives us a new opportunity and a second chance to start over. If we change our perception about who we are and what we can accomplish and if we remember the power we have to overcome the obstacles before us, equipped with the truth, we can overcome fear. We can rid ourselves of the things that habitually remind us of our worst failures, countless disappointments, deepest regrets, and weakest moments.

We can be strong and courageous—ruled by our most hopeful thoughts, our greatest successes, and our grandest opportunities.

Masters in Disguise

Throughout the long journey, the entire assembly of Israelites continued to regret their decision to leave Egypt. *"If only we had died in Egypt or in this desert. Or in this wilderness! Why is the Lord bringing us to this land only to let us fall by the sword? Our wives and children will be taken as plunder. Wouldn't it be better for us to go back to Egypt? We should choose a leader and go back..."* Numbers 14:2-4.

Even though their former way of life was brutal for the Israelites, every time they realized their comforts had been compromised they wanted to go back to the old way of life.

They often sought to replace their leadership with new leaders, and on one occasion they chose to abandon the leadership of God and Moses and return to the idols of Egypt. They threw all their valuables into the fire, and fashioned a golden calf.

There will always be a tendency to want to go back to the old. For us, going back often means returning to our old habits or returning to food. We jeopardize our own advancement unconsciously by sabotaging ourselves. We "go back" by choosing another addiction. In the bariatric world this is referred to as "*transfer or crossover addiction.*"

According to Dr. Lance Dodes, assistant clinical professor of psychiatry at Harvard Medical School and the author of *Breaking Addiction*, it is not unusual for recovering addicts to transfer one obsession to another. "*It's been well known for a very long time that A.A. meetings used to be filled with smoke because people shifted their focus from drinking to cigarettes. Alcoholism isn't about alcohol any more than compulsive gambling is about playing roulette—or winning money. Addiction is a solution to an emotional need. If you deprive someone of one solution to their emotional problems, it's not surprising that they'll find another one instead.*"

For many of us, food has been our addiction. When we leave food behind, we seek another. Smoking, drinking, shopping, gambling, and even over-exercising can be dangerous substitutes for overeating and develop into transfer addictions. Even the thrill of losing weight can become an addiction. But soon we find that these don't satisfy. They are as useless as a golden calf.

You may find that, like myself, you have used food to cover up a lifetime of pain and disappointments. If you have been here, you're not alone. Most patients have been there at one time or another—and so have I.

The story of the Israelites closely parallels my own. Somewhere in my past, I had left one place of famine behind and tried to fill it with another. Food had become my Pharaoh. It offered to satisfy my inward hungers and successfully lured me astray with promises of fulfillment. What was meant to nourish and strengthen me eventually began to enslave me. I didn't realize it so much at the time, but I was trying to avoid facing painful situations of the past. I believed food was what I needed to fill those empty and hurting places. I relied on it to give me temporary relief and fill my emotional deficits. And it worked—for a while.

When we are no longer depending on food to cover the pain, it is inevitable that life's hurts will once again begin to stir. What

> *"... Addiction is a solution to an emotional need. If you deprive someone of one solution to their emotional problems, it's not surprising that they'll find another one instead."*

then? If we have not made adjustments towards recovery, the voids that are left will only require more medication. We must be aware of the tendency to go back or turn to another comfort at any time. Like an army chasing behind us in hot pursuit, unwilling to let us go, our former rulers hold fast, sabotaging our every attempt to free ourselves, seeking to bring us back under their dominion.

There were many times during the years after my surgery when life became extremely stressful and held life-changing events. My mother broke her hip, and with her failing memory continuing to threaten her well-being, my sister and I had to make the decision to move her from her home of 60 years and place her in a skilled nursing care facility. Her loss of memory meant a painful loss of the relationship for us. There were nights full of wakefulness, tears, and hours filled with sadness.

It was during these times that I thought it would have been so easy to return to self-medication to find relief. There were moments when I wanted to reach for food or another substitute.

We are tempted to imagine that going back would be safer, easier, and more comfortable than going forward, but that is not true. The ills of obesity and slavery to addictions are not safe, easy, or comfortable, they are life-threatening. We must be careful what we believe to be true. Even though we know these paths hold temporary and short-lived promises of reprieve, none of them can reach deep enough into the soul to erase the agony we feel. Just as with other addictions, food addiction is not about food, and going back will not be our answer. Food and other dependences do not offer us true solutions. The issue is much deeper and we must be careful not to silence it.

When we constantly feed our feelings with food, or seek other ways to fill the voids, instead of learning how to lay them aside, they only become unnecessary baggage that drags us down, mentally as well as physically. They become explosive disasters waiting to happen.

Food and fad diets may have deceived us with false promises to save, but they will never be enough to redeem us from our past mistakes, deliver us from our distresses, fill our inward hungers, or cure us of our addictions. They will always fall short and leave us surrounded by an army of defeat, depression, and emptiness. That is, if we let them.

The Israelites were right about one thing; before they could enter into the new land they would need a new leader. Moses had led the people out of slavery, but another leader would need to lead them into their new home. Likewise, I needed to be under the direction of new leadership. My emotional hungers may have led me into obesity. Weight loss surgery may have served to lead me out, giving me the opportunity to successfully lose weight and regain my health, but this was not the Promised Land for which I was searching. Surgery alone didn't fix the underlying issues. I needed to find a more permanent solution to carry me into long-term success.

My journey has been more than losing weight. It has been more than making an effort to change old eating habits or even replacing old thinking patterns, although these were extremely important. It has been a search to find what was holding me back from being free from addictions—a journey to discover what brought me to the land of captivity in the first place and how to sever its ties once and for all.

We may inadvertently bring the rulers from our past with us, but we can find freedom. We can choose to find the solutions that will produce changes for the long-term.

As we circle through this maintenance phase, it will be important to eliminate anything that may jeopardize our success or our ability to live successfully in the new land. We can choose to leave the old behind, be willing to get to the root cause, and be ready to make the mindset changes needed to carry us forward. We can make sure that we continue to identify the rulers of our past, and not let them rule over our present—for if they do, they will also rule our future.

Every kingdom has a ruler. Isn't it time to choose another? *"Who or what will we choose to lead us into our Promised Land?"*

"Who or what will we allow to rule us now?"

PART FIVE:

Into the Promised Land

Maintenance and Beyond

**Then you will know the truth,
and the truth will set you free.**

John 8:32

Thrown For A Loop

Rain! whose soft architectural hands have power to cut stones, and chisel to shapes of grandeur the very mountains.

Henry Ward Beecher

Sometimes the storms of life are more like passing showers, there's not much to them; and we find ourselves none-the-worse after they pass. Sure, it may have rained on our parade, but life still goes on.

And then there are the larger storms. The cracks of thunder are definitely loud enough to stir you from your deepest dreams. The rain is falling at a rate far beyond our ability to recover. The water is rising, and suddenly we are in over our head. Where do we turn?

Three years after surgery, I had lost 164 pounds, I was maintaining my weight loss, and I was walking 3 to 6 miles a day. I even had this great idea to sign up for a 1/2 marathon and was just getting ready to train with a local group for a walk at one of my long-dreamed of destinations in Kiawah Island, SC.

But, suddenly, I found myself in the middle of a raging storm. Totally unexpected, this storm arose in spite of my excitement (actually, in the middle of it). It was stronger than I expected. Like a hurricane that didn't want to move on, it stalled in its place, wreaking havoc and lowering my defenses. This storm wasn't about eating habits, weight loss, discipline, or even weight gain. It came in the form of hypoglycemia, and although it was a physical issue, it was taking a toll on my emotional state.

There is a 2.5 mile walking track in the center of Wrightsville Beach, NC, known to all the locals as *"The Loop."* The smells of salty ocean air and melodious suntan lotions dance their way among the busy plethora of activity—people, dogs, bikes, and baby strollers. So, whether you prefer walking, running, or just making your way to the beach with an armful of towels, umbrellas, surfboards, sand buckets, beach balls, and picnics—you'll feel right at home.

As you make your way across one of two bridges that stretch across the Intracoastal Waterway to the island, there are rich, beautiful marshlands and the sidewalk winds over Banks Channel, around through the main street just a block away from the ocean—giving it that small town atmosphere with little shops and seafood fare. On occasion, the local churches along the route will offer a bottle of iced water and a smile. It just makes one thankful to live at the beach. This walk is as healing to the soul as it is to the body.

And then it happened. For several days in a row, I couldn't make it halfway around the loop without the symptoms of low blood sugar. It threw me *for a loop* all right. I was in trouble. Being totally unprepared, I had no food with me, and although I passed by several restaurants and a local grocery, I had no money to purchase any. I spotted several police cars, but not knowing exactly what was happening to me, I really couldn't justify asking for help. I kept looking at people's faces as they passed, trying to decide if anyone cared enough to sacrifice their walk to help someone who was about to hit the curb. I was confused and close to fainting. I finally made it to my car, located my purse, drove to the first fast-food restaurant just over the bridge to the mainland, and ordered a burger.

For over a year I struggled to correct the issue myself, but to no avail. I sought help from my surgeon, my family doctor, and my endocrinologist. Each one referred to me to a dietitian and I followed their advice. I knew how to follow the rules. That was something I could do, but the rules weren't working. There seemed to be nothing to relieve the symptoms and as time passed, I grew worse. I felt as though I was circling back to where I started. Unable to get my hypoglycemia under control, I began struggling with weight regain. Physical activity, workouts in the gym, along with my daily walks, came to an end. I had to abandon, or at least postpone, my dream of walking in the half-marathon at Kiawah.

I was told of another nutritional counselor who might be able to help, so I made an appointment. After several visits, she agreed that dietary modifications weren't enough to correct the problem. She recommended a specialist in the area who had experience dealing with RNY patients who were experiencing hypoglycemia. So I made an appointment.

After several tests, it was confirmed. I was diagnosed with severe post-surgical hypoglycemia and was handed a prescription medication that might help. On the one hand, I was relieved. Someone had been able to give me an answer, diagnose my problems, and in addition, they offered me a medication that could help alleviate my symptoms. It was an answer to prayer and an opportunity to return to living a normal life again—the life I had earned.

But, prescription drugs? I had seen it coming, but when I actually held the prescription in my hand, I was devastated. The thing I had feared was now upon me. Prescriptions were the last thing I wanted. I had surgery to avoid them. I had worked so hard to get off all my medication, and going back on them seemed like a move in the wrong direction. I had followed all of the rules. I had stayed within the limits. I had eaten right and I had been faithful to exercise. But, the rules had failed me. This was certainly not the way I had imaged life after surgery would turn out. My faith in the process had been shaken to its core. It seemed my hope for a normal life and everything I had worked for was being swept away. What now?

CHAPTER 32

Standing at the Gateway

**"For you are about to cross the Jordan to go in
to possess the land which the LORD your God is
giving you,and you shall possess it and live in it,"**
Deuteronomy 11:31 (NASB)

I have heard it said that triumphs follow trials and trials follow triumphs. Just when you think you have arrived and it's time to celebrate, you realize there is another test coming your way. My newfound health problems were that kind of moment.

I once thought that the Promised Land was the restoration of my body and my health, but I was beginning to realize that it wasn't. Like the Israelites, I had come a long way. I had crossed my own vast desert, ridding myself of excess baggage, shedding old mindsets and letting go of limiting beliefs. But, not only was I not in the Promised Land, there were other thoughts running through my head.

This crisis had also brought with it serious contemplation. It caused me to question if I had made the right decision to have the surgery in the first place or if I should consider having a reversal. It made me question what I really wanted. I wondered what it would take to possess the Promised Land or if I would I ever get there.

For the Israelites, the time had come—the moment they had been anticipating for over forty years. God announced it was time to move into the Promised Land. They were going home—home to the land that had been promised to them by God since the days of Abraham.

The pilgrimage to Canaan had not been an easy one. They had been fighting battles just to get to the border of the Promised Land. Just as they waited to cross over, God presented them with a choice. As they stood in a valley between two mountains, Mt Gerizim and Mt Ebal, they were reminded of what they had experienced since their escape from Egypt. They were told what success in the new land would demand and what it would require to dwell there. They had a decision to make. Just as in their decision to leave Egypt years before, it would be a decision of life or death.

No matter what they would choose, God was clear. There would be more battles to fight. Some of the tribes decided to settle here, on the east side of the Jordan River, and others chose to journey on to live in the land of Canaan. But no matter where they chose to live, they would all enter into the Promised Land and conquer the enemies together.

Here at the oasis of Kadesh-Barnea, this new generation paused to consider their decision to travel across the Jordan River and on into Canaan.

Imagine standing on the border of the Promised Land, on the edge of the Jordan River. You have come such a long way. You have been freed from slavery, escaped a pursuing Pharaoh, crossed the Red Sea, wandered in a hostile desert for forty years, fought numerous battles, and now you're almost there. And even though there is another river to cross and a few more battles to wage, the logical decision is to press forward. God has promised to fight their battles for them and with God on their side they can't lose. With a fertile land flowing with every good thing within their reach, how could they even consider not going forward? How could they consider turning down the opportunity to live there? But, logic has very little to do with how one feels when in the middle of a life-changing crisis.

At this moment, I found myself in the same dilemma. I had come such a long way, and I was so close, but I was struggling with the same decision. I was tired and weary from fighting so many battles. Facing this ensuing battle with unpredictable insulin levels, I was tempted to turn back. Learning that I had to go back on medication literally shook my world. I believed that once I had the surgery, followed the rules, and practiced compliance, things would work out just fine. But that didn't seem to be the case. It was as if I was being swept away by a raging flood, leaving me nowhere to stand—or so I thought.

CHAPTER 33

The Walls Come Tumbling Down

By faith the walls of Jericho fell...
Hebrews 11:30

Just like the Israelites, we too, have a choice to make. Once we are out of Egypt, we can choose to stop and "settle" before we reach the full potential of what our passage has to offer, or we can move forward and occupy our Promised Land.

For the Israelites, the entrance into the Promised Land began with a walk of faith, and their possession of the land was accompanied by miracles and wonders beyond their imagination. Once they neared the border, they had to cross the Jordan River. The Jordan is a natural barrier between the arid desert wilderness and the fertile country of Canaan. Just like the Red Sea, the Jordan River represented the separation between the old way of life and the new. And just like the Red Sea, it looked as if it would be impossible to cross because the river was at flood stage.

The Israelites had grown to know and trust God more and more during their journey to the Promised Land. They had trusted God during the battles to defeat their enemies, but as they entered into the land they had to trust Him from yet another dimension of faith.

Instead of simply parting the waters for the Israelites as God had done at the Red Sea, they had to trust that He would see them through to the other side. The water of the Jordan River didn't part until the Israelites actually put their feet into the water at the rivers edge.

Led by Joshua, God miraculously opened the way for the Israelites to cross the Jordan River and enter into the land of Canaan. They were ready to possess the land, but possession would depend on their ability to see themselves for who they really were, their willingness to fight for what is rightfully theirs, and their readiness to trust God.

In other words, there were still battles to fight. The Israelites had to deal with the "giants in the land." The giants had to be driven out, and God had a plan and a promise to make it happen. Failure to follow His plan and wage those remaining necessary battles would set them up for trouble in the long-term. God said, *"....they will become snares and traps for you, whips on your backs and thorns in your eyes, until you perish from this good land...." Joshua 23:13.*

Their first battle was at Jericho. Humanly speaking, it was logically impossible for the Israelites to win a battle against Jericho. It was an indestructible stronghold, a massive fortress. With it's enormous walls, giant-size inhabitants, and horrible leaders, it was impenetrable. Two walls surrounded the six-acre town. One wall was six feet thick and about 20 to 26 feet high. Between those two massive walls was a ditch nine feet deep and 27 feet wide, which was cut through solid rock. Another wall stood about 46 feet above ground level outside the retaining wall.

On their own, they could never conquer it. No amount of physical strength or mental strategy could bring it down. God revealed His plan. He told Joshua to march around the city once every day for six days with seven priests carrying ram's horns in front of an ark, which represented the Presence of God. On the seventh day they were to march around the city seven times without speaking a word. The only sound would be the sound of the priests blowing their horns. Then Joshua was to order the people to shout and the walls of the city would collapse, allowing the Israelites to charge straight into the city and destroy it.

Really? That was God's plan? Just walk around the city seven times and the walls would fall? It seemed crazy. Logically, it made no sense at all. The Israelites had to trust that their victory at Jericho would be won—not with worldly weapons, but with supernatural ones.

I had escaped obesity through the miracle of bariatric surgery; I had traveled through an emotional desert, working to shed old mindsets and old labels; I had waged battles against food addiction, emotional eating, and more; but now I was standing in front of a giant fortress of my own. Hypoglycemia and a return to prescription medication was my Jericho. I had no idea how I would ever move past it.

Then, while on the way to the pharmacy to fill my prescription medication, I received a phone call that proved to be much more than an ordinary phone call. It was actually a wake-up call from God. It came in the form of an invitation from a close friend and pastor. I was invited to be a speaker at a workshop for a church. The name of the church: Reimage. Coincidence? I think not. But it was the conference theme that really got my attention: *"Unshakable!"*

"Wait just one minute, Lord. I am in the middle of a storm, I am teetering on the verge of collapse both physically and emotionally, my world is crumbling around me and I'm questioning the strength of my footing, and you want me to tell others that while everything around us crumbles, we are standing on unshakable ground?"

There it was, the loud crack of thunder that went rumbling through my very being. It was the sound I needed to regain my resolve. It had reminded me that the ground on which I stood WAS a firm foundation, the kind that holds up under the worst of storms. Just as the Israelites had followed Joshua into another kingdom, more than 30 years before, I made the decision to follow God's Truth by placing my trust in His unconditional love for me. I had chosen to believe that God's Word is true. I had been spiritually re-born, choosing to live in God's unshakable Kingdom. But suddenly I realized I wasn't living from that truth.

Hungry for The Truth, Filled By the Promise

I had worked to change my body. I had worked to change my thinking. But now, it was becoming clear that God was doing some work within my heart.

Just as with weight loss surgery, this journey wasn't a spontaneous event. I may have awakened from surgery physically transformed in some ways, but I didn't wake up 164 pounds thinner. Likewise, my spiritual "aha" moments were not huge Red Sea miracles, but rather subtle spiritual shifts that were the simplest, yet, the biggest shifts of all.

There is a metaphor that our life's journey is like going around a mountain. Although we circle back to the same landmarks, each time around, we experience them from a different perspective, with a higher understanding. I was, indeed, making another loop, *little by little* and *lap by lap*, until I increased enough to possess the land.

"Walking with God" is the practice of applying Christian principles and beliefs to everyday life. Much like circling the desert, or circling the walls of Jericho, this is a walk that happens many times. Throughout our lives, God continues to reveal Himself to us in a deeper way. We circle God's truth time and time again, continually renewing our awareness of who He is, what He did, what we have in Christ, who He is in us, and who we are in Him.

> There is a difference in knowing something and actually applying its truth to your life.

There is a difference in knowing something and actually applying its truth to your life. During this phase of my journey, God began to remind me of the truths that I already knew about Him, but there was something more. There was more knowledge to be gained. There were things God wanted me to experience.

When our story of the Israelites began, the Pharaoh was not only holding them in bondage, but he had increased their suffering and demanded the impossible. Then Moses announced that God would come to their rescue. By all outward appearances, God's attempt to save them was only making things worse.

Moses inquired of the Lord, asking the same question we often ask during our trials and hardships in life, "*Why, Lord, why have you brought trouble on this people? Is this why you sent me? Ever since I went to Pharaoh to speak in your name, he has brought trouble on this people, and you have not rescued your people at all.*" God's answer is recorded in *Exodus 6:3. "God also spoke to Moses and said to him: "I am the Lord. I appeared to Abraham, Isaac, and Jacob as God Almighty, but by my name 'The Lord' I did not make myself known to them. I also established my covenant with them, to give them the land of Canaan, the land in which they resided as aliens.*"

God didn't just promise to deliver the Israelites from Egypt and give them the land of Canaan for their own, He also promised to reveal Himself to them—that they might *know* Him. The Israelites knew *about* God. Their forefathers, Abraham, Isaac, and Jacob knew God as the Mighty God, Creator, the Judge of the Heavens and the Earth—their provider and keeper.

They also knew God's name was "*The Lord,*" the God of grace and mercy. Even though they were holding on to a promise that God would deliver them from Egypt, the Children of the Promise had never personally experienced God's grace and mercy for themselves. They had never experienced firsthand the fulfilling of the promises He had made to them. They knew *about* him, but they didn't *know* Him by personal experience. It was only after the Exodus, when God fulfilled His promise, did they come to know the One True and Living God, the One who keeps His Promises. They came to know through experience His personal and unconditional love, intimate care, unlimited favor, and personal redemption.

God brought the Israelites out of Egypt. He took them as His own, to bring them into a relationship with Himself. He delivered them from slavery, parted the sea, and brought them to Mt. Sinai to reveal Himself to them. There He gave them the Ten Commandments, but these weren't just a list of Do's and Don'ts, it was a means by which they could come to know Him.

But the commandments weren't all He gave them. At the same time, He also presented the Israelites with a blueprint to build a tabernacle. It was a place where they could meet with Him face-to-face, a place where His Presence could dwell among them.

In the wilderness, they had to learn to trust God to meet their physical needs. From the time the Israelites left Egypt until the time they reached The Promised Land, He had fed them manna—Bread from Heaven—for more than forty years. During their journey they had learned to trust him physically, emotionally, and spiritually; they had come to recognize Him as the Bread of Life, the One who could meet all of their needs. But once they reached the Promised Land, the manna ended. Entering the Promised Land meant they could rest in God's abundant provision, and know fulfillment at last.

My "unshakable" phone call was a kind of face-to-face moment with God, a moment when I realized I wasn't fully living out of God's truth. As a Christian, I knew I belonged to Him, but I needed to be reminded of who I was. I realized that God was orchestrating my journey to ultimately bring *me* closer to Him.

God had rescued me out of the land of obesity, delivered me from physical slavery, and given me back my health. Then, I had achieved emotional freedom by learning how to tear down the lies of the past, uncover the present truth, and win the battle of my mind. Now, He was beginning to restore areas in my spiritual life.

I had known God as my Deliverer for decades. I knew God loved me. I knew He had purchased my peace, carried my shame, healed me, and set me free. But, now, I realized that this was another lap around that mountain. God had designed this journey so that I might experience Him in these areas like never before.

He was urging me to "take up residence in the new land." When I started looking beyond my physical and emotional deliverance from obesity, I allowed myself to experience God's redemption in a whole new dimension.

As I trusted God to lead the way, I discovered freedom from shame and fear and I found more inner healing. Embracing God's love and grace was a process that strengthened my spiritual identity. It taught me how to dwell in a place of greater spiritual freedom and deeper self-worth.

But just because I had discovered how to dwell in the Promised Land did not mean there wouldn't be battles to fight. As I crossed over into this new territory, God began to teach me how to win the spiritual battles in my life.

No Ordinary Weapons

In ancient times, a fortress was called a stronghold. They were built to secure newfound territories. They were also built with the intent to keep the enemy out, but they also served to keep those who lived there in. Before the Israelites could live in the Promised Land, they had to tear down the strongholds within the land and rid themselves of its inhabitants.

When we hold fast and strong to our beliefs, they become strongholds. When our beliefs are false, it can prevent the truth from coming in. They can hold us captive with false impressions, misguided fears, and uncertainties. The Battle of Jericho became a blue print for how I could tear down the strongholds of my life and let God be my Stronghold.

Jericho represented my truth, with all its misconceptions or past perceptions that were no longer relevant. These strongholds needed to come down. I needed to replace my truth for God's truth. His truth needed to rule over my circumstances.

So, how do we tear down those walls, and replace our strongholds with God's truth? These battles are fought in the mind. Just like I learned to bring my mind and body into agreement, winning spiritual battles required overthrowing the lies that ruled my thinking and allowed the truth to dominate. *2 Corinthians 10:4-5* tells us how. *"The weapons we fight with are not the weapons of the world. On the contrary, they have divine power to demolish strongholds. We demolish arguments and every pretension that sets itself up against the knowledge of God, and we take captive every thought to make it obedient to Christ."*

> Just like I learned to bring my mind and body into agreement, winning spiritual battles required overthrowing the lies that ruled my thinking and allowed the truth to dominate.

Armed for Battle: God's way of fighting battles looks nothing like our own; His battle plan is simple. *"The weapons we fight with are not the weapons of the world. On the contrary, they have divine power to demolish strongholds."* God has equipped us with spiritual weapons, which have the power we need to demolish strongholds. Spiritual battles require no worldly weapons, little physical effort, and no mental strategy, but rather a walk of faith, a knowledge of God and His Word, and a willingness to exchange our truth for His.

Circle the Fortress: How do we identify our untrue beliefs or strongholds? Consider what you believe about your circumstances. What do you believe about yourself? What is your truth? What are the thoughts you have been telling yourself?

My reaction to my diagnosis of post-surgical hypoglycemia was based on my own beliefs. *"This is hopeless. I did all of this work for nothing. Why did I ever have this surgery in the first place? I'm no better off than I was before. Going back on medication means that I'm right back where I started. I'm a failure."*

Walk in His Truth: *"We demolish arguments and every pretension that sets itself up against the knowledge of God…"* What declarations are you making about your life? Are they false claims (or pretensions)? Are they supported by God's Word? Is your truth in agreement or disagreement with God's Truth?

The next part of this verse says, *"we take captive every thought to make it obedient to Christ."* We take our thoughts captive by not letting them dominate us, but instead, we rule over them.

What is God's truth? What does God say about the situation? Does He say it's hopeless? Did He label me a failure, or an overcomer? Did I consider that He was on my side, fighting on my behalf? Was I trusting Him as my Deliverer?

The word *obedient* means to come into agreement. I had to take a good look at my beliefs. My truth didn't agree with what I knew to be true about God. It didn't agree with His Word. My truth was ruling over God's truth. My claims were unsupported, leaving me on shaky ground. Was I really right back where I started? Did I weigh 302 pounds again? Had I not been delivered from diabetes, high blood pressure, and other ailments? Did taking prescription medications mean I hadn't reached success?

God's truth *silenced* the untrue thoughts of my circumstances and my self-talk. When I discovered the truth about God, it demolished the false evidence and revealed the genuine. In order to win the battle of the mind, I had to train my thoughts to agree with God's Word. When I compared my truth to God's truth, I found that my claims were false. They didn't agree with what God says about my circumstances or about me. My situation was not hopeless and I was not a failure.

God's Word is not just ink on the pages of a book. We can follow Him as He leads us into victory. His power can dwell within us, satisfy our inward needs, and give us the ability and the power to *will and to act* according to His intended purpose. When our inward needs are satisfied, it gives us the power to be compliant.

Just as the Israelites followed Joshua, we can follow Jesus Christ. Jesus is the Truth. He is the Living Word. He is God in person—powerful, alive, and active and His Holy Spirit will lead us into all truth. His Truth can rule our lives.

Let The Walls Fall: Just like circling the walls of Jericho, I found victory when I began to uncover the false truths or strongholds in my life and exchange them for God's truth. This allowed me to live out my new life in a place of freedom and peace.

He Loves Us Out

Do you *know* the Lord? Are you walking in agreement with His truth? There is more to knowing God than just knowing *about* Him.

God brought the Israelites out of slavery and chose them to be His people because He loved them. And just like the Israelites, God has chosen you to be His treasured possession, too. When you call on Him, He comes to your rescue. He will bring you out of the land of slavery because of His great love for you.

Like manna in the wilderness, we all hunger for the same things in our lives: unconditional love and acceptance, security, peace, and significance. God is the only one who can offer us what we are really hungry for—He is the bread of life. He satisfies our thirsty souls and fills our hungry hearts. God's love for you is unfathomable, unconditional, extravagant, without end, and beyond measure.

You, too, stand on the brink of a new land. Just like the Israelites, God offers you the same opportunity to choose Him, to experience freedom, to begin anew, to embrace a new identity, and to dwell in a new place.

He has already prepared the way of escape. He stands ready to fight your battles, to heal you from your diseases, to give you new life, and a chance to live it to the fullest. By exchanging your truth for His, your strongholds will crumble and fall and God will become your Life and your Stronghold.

Have you experienced firsthand the unconditional love and unmerited grace He offers? He is waiting to reveal His truth and His love—and all you have to do is ask.

When I prayed to see the fulfillment of my Promised Land, God heard my prayer and He was faithful. He brought me out of the land of slavery. Only after my exodus could I truly *know* Him and experience His love and His deliverance more fully. I found the physical, emotional, and spiritual increase and freedom I was seeking. Possessing the Promised Land means dwelling in these truths—*living* out of who God says I am. I was home, at last.

CHAPTER 34

Welcome Home

**For He satisfies the longing soul and
fills the hungry soul with good.**

Psalm 107:9 (AMP)

It was time for my 4-year, annual RNY checkup. My blood work
had significantly improved and I'd even lost a few pounds since
last year's visit. Nothing to fear. Right? So, why was I stressed?

That morning as I stepped on the scale, following my daily
routine, I was five pounds heavier than the previous week. What
happened? Surely, I didn't gain five pounds in a week. Not this
week. Of all days, did it have to be today? This was the day when my
surgeon would evaluate my progress over the last year. Suddenly
the panic of weight regain started to set in.

I had a flashback to that 302-pound moment when I moved
the weight on the scale past the dreaded 300 mark. For an
instant, all of those old feelings started to return. My mind
reverted to the old habits and tricks of the past. How could I lose
five pounds in five minutes? As I stood in the closet, I started
to consider my options. Did I need to change my outfit, take off
some jewelry, or find lighter shoes?

Then I stopped. I took a good look in the mirror. And a
miracle happened. No, I didn't miraculously lose those five
pounds. I realized that the number on the scale wasn't telling
the whole truth.

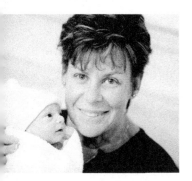

Gavin (June 2007)

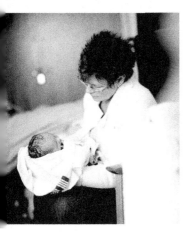

Genevieve (April 2012)

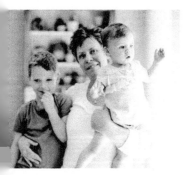

Gavin and Genevieve (2013)

Yes, I had gained back a few pounds, but my success wasn't just about the physical alone, it was more about the transformation within. My miracle was the realization that my weight did not define my failure or my success. My success wasn't based on a number, a certain dress size, or even a perfect bill of health. True success is so much bigger than that. It comes from a contentment deep within. Possessing my promise entails knowing God more intimately and discovering who I am in the light of that knowledge. My success is based on who I am on the inside.

It's been eight years since I had weight loss surgery. Although I had gained from my lowest weight, those few pounds did not change my health or my quality of life, just my clothing size. Physically, I'm healthy and active. Even though I've had my share of set backs and I still have to work my way through a few battles from time to time, losing weight has given me my life back. I am no longer a slave to food or obesity.

As I stand firmly planted in this good land, I pray that I will never forget where I came from. Although I still have sleep apnea and I still battle symptoms of hypoglycemia, I am free from life-threatening diseases such as high blood pressure, diabetes, and high cholesterol—diseases that would have shortened my life. My doctor says I most likely had hypoglycemia all along and that my weight, diet, and eating habits could have been masking the symptoms. Currently, I am taking a medication, which is helping normalize my blood sugar levels. I was also placed back on thyroid medication, which has not only improved my health, but has helped to lessen my hypoglycemia and sleep apnea. Even with this huge unexpected consequence of hypoglycemia and even though I still have sleep apnea, I can say that I'm glad I had the surgery and I'm embracing my new life, my new body, and the new me.

Emotionally, I am living in a new place. Living in the Promised Land doesn't mean that my battles are over, it just means that now I'm physically, emotionally, and spiritually equipped to confront the challenges that seemed insurmountable before. On occasion, I still find myself looking for something to eat when I'm not hungry, but because I know how to deal with the inside issues, food has taken its rightful place. I've learned that I can enjoy guilt-free, healthy eating. In fact, I love and appreciate food more than ever. I have also lost most of the pounds I had regained.

Best of all, my new lap is getting lots of practice. In 2012, we were blessed with the arrival of our second grandchild—a little girl named Genevieve. In 2013, two more little ones made their way into our family, into our hearts, and into my lap. A little boy named Finn and a little girl named Saylor.

God was faithful to His promise. He brought me out of the land of obesity, but He didn't bring me out to wander around in a wilderness. Coming out of obesity is wonderful, but that's not the end. He brought me out so that He might bring me into a new place—a place of life and freedom. He brought me out because He loved me. He brought me out to bring me closer to Himself. As He continues to show me more of His extravagant love and mercy, the more freedom I possess.

More importantly, during this experience I have changed from the inside out. I have learned more about what it means to live in God's unshakable kingdom. I am living out of a deeper spiritual truth—a deeper awareness of who I am. I found the ultimate place of success and inward satisfaction—a deeper and more intimate knowledge of God—a satisfaction that fills every longing, meets every need, is uniquely fitted, personally individualized, and completely tailor-made. It satisfies the body, soul, and spirit. I have possessed the promise. Little by little I increased enough to possess the Land. I'm living my life with a greater expectation of the continuing wonders God has prepared for me.

Many years before the Israelites reached the Promised Land, Abraham stood near the plains of the Jordan. He was leaving one life behind and turning his eyes toward the land God would give to his offspring. Before him he could see the spacious land with lush, well-watered gardens, a place that held broad promises in every direction. It was time to move forward, to possess the land of Canaan, to claim what had been promised to him. God whispered

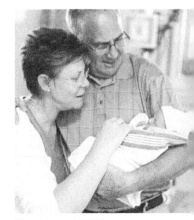

Finn (August 2013)

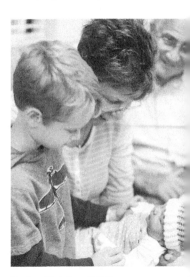

Saylor (October 2013)

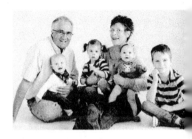

Grandkids (2014)

to Abraham. *"Lift up your eyes now and look from the place where you are, for all the land which you can see...(is yours)...arise and walk...."* Genesis 13:14,17 (NKJV).

You, too, stand in the gateway of a new land—a new kingdom. Just as with the Israelites, your journey there will not be easy. There will be battles, tests, and trials.

In ancient times, when warriors were called to battle, they were assembled together. The officers who stood alongside them informed them of the dangers and painful reality of war and what was waiting on the battlefield. They were also reminded of the joy of winning and the glories of victory. They were exhorted and encouraged to stand firm and tall, to throw back their shoulders and look the enemy straight on, eyeball to eyeball, and courageously face the battle ahead.

This is the message I leave with you. No matter which side of surgery you are on, overcoming obesity is an epic adventure with many long and difficult battles. I know the struggle; I've lived it. At times, you will feel the like a stranger in the new land. It will be difficult to break free from the things that hold you to the past. In the beginning, some days will be difficult, long, and seemingly endless. Like the Israelites, you will grow tired and long to return to the safety of the familiar.

But I am here to tell you that you can make it. You, too, can claim the promise of physical, emotional, and spiritual freedom. Beyond the battles and the despair of the desert, there are new joys that lie ahead.

Lift up your eyes. Look from the place where you stand and gaze into the future. Can you see it? It's there. Your Promised Land is waiting. It's been prepared for you. It's everything you could ask for and more. When you get there, you'll *know* it—a place of peace, restoration, and fulfillment—a place you can call home. It is a land that gives you the opportunity to exchange death for life. It is a good land. A land of riches where there is no lack—and your deepest hungers are satisfied. A place where you can exchange His life and Truth for yours and you can live out of who God says you are. You are not who you think you are—you are so much more. You, too, can experience God's love and all that He has for you in a land flowing with blessings beyond measure.

It's *your* time to arise and walk—out of the land of obesity and into *your* Promised Land.

"We were slaves of Pharaoh in Egypt, but the Lord brought us out of Egypt with

a mighty hand. Before our eyes the Lord sent signs and wonders—great and

terrible—on Egypt and Pharaoh and his whole household. But he brought us out

from there to bring us in and give us the land he promised..."

Deuteronomy 6:21-23

"But it was because the Lord loved you and kept the oath that he swore to your

ancestors, that He brought you out with a mighty hand and redeemed you from

the land of slavery and from the power of Pharaoh king of Egypt"

Deuteronomy 7:8

"Now to Him who is able to do immeasurably more than all we

ask or imagine, according to His power that is at work within us,

to Him be the glory... .for ever and ever."

Ephesians 3:20-21

Praise for
Out Of Obesity and into the Promised Land

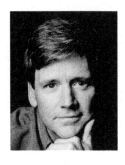

"Julia Holloman has done her homework! She takes readers on an inspiring and informative journey while highlighting the guidelines and lifestyle changes required to successfully maintain weight loss. Her personable, easy-to-read account from a patient's perspective is sure to help others enjoy the success that Julia has achieved. I recommend this book to healthcare providers, patients, and anyone considering bariatric surgery."

—David R. Miles, M.D., Bariatric Surgeon, Miles Surgical, Wilmington, NC

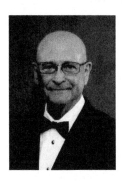

"In Out of Obesity, the reader experiences the extensive physical, mental, emotional, and spiritual journey on which the bariatric surgery patient embarks. This journey begins well before the operation, and never truly has an end. In weight loss and comorbidity improvement, success is dependent on the patient, the surgeon and a multidisciplinary team working in concert over the long term.

As Julia Holloman shares her journey, she provides valuable information and insight that will benefit those who are considering bariatric surgery, those who have already had the procedure, and the family and friends providing support to both. She demonstrates the importance of educating yourself thoroughly prior to surgery and exploring your treatment options with a trusted, caring professional who is committed to your safety and success."

—Dr. Neil E. Hutcher, Chief Medical Officer, Surgical Review Corporation

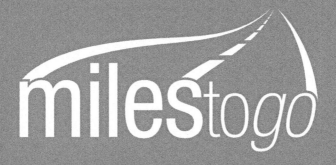

For ongoing support visit

WWW.MILESTOGOBLOG.COM

JULIA HOLLOMAN
certified bariatric coach, bcbu
certified bariatric support group leader

offering education and encouragement
for weight loss surgery success

Made in the USA
Columbia, SC
04 September 2021

44895647R00189